Bircher-Benner Manuals

Manual for patients with liver and gallbladder conditions

The latest biophysically scientific insights on life energy,
food energy and the effects of fresh raw fruit and vegetable food.
Comprehensive instructions for the application and preparation
of the vegetable raw-food diet according to Bircher-Benner.
Menus and recipes from the Medical Centre Bircher-Benner,
CH-8784 Braunwald

Dr med. Andres A. Bircher
and employees of the Bircher-Benner Medical Center
Lilli Bircher, Anne-Cecile Bircher and Pascal Bircher

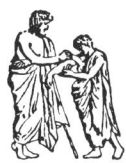

EDITION BIRCHER-BENNER
CH-8784 BRAUNWALD

Bircher-Benner Manuals

1. Manual for patients with multiple sclerosis and degenerative nervous diseases
2. Manual for patients with liver and gallbladder conditions
3. Manual for families and children
4. Manual of fresh juices, raw vegetables and fruit dishes
5. Manual for improvement of the immune system and against susceptibility to infection
6. Manual for mountaineers and athletes
7. Manual for diabetics
8. Manual for support and preventive therapy for lung diseases
9. Enjoy food without table salt
10. Manual for patients with rheumatism and arthritis
11. Manual for men with prostate conditions
12. Manual for patients with kidney and bladder conditions
13. Manual for venous diseases
14. Manual for patients with gastrointestinal conditions
15. Manual for nutrition during pregnancy and lactation
16. Manual for gynaecological problems and menopause
17. Manual for the prevention of cancer and accompanying therapies
18. Manual for headache and migraine
19. Manual for patients with hypertension, cardiovascular disease and arteriosclerosis
20. Manual for overcoming anxiety and depression
21. Manual for patients with skin diseases or sensitive skin
22. Manual for persons suffering from stress
23. Manual for persons suffering from allergies
24. Manual for prevention of dementia and Alzheimer's disease
25. Manual for internal treatment of eye problems
26. Manual for treatment of weight problems, overweight, and anorexia

These manuals take into consideration the results of global research, the development of the art and science of medicine over more than a century and the experience of the renowned Bircher-Benner Klinik. The reader will feel the helpful support of the well-informed physician at every step of the way.

32rd edition 2015, revised and enlarged. Translated from the original German.

All rights, including the right of reproduction in excerpts, photomechanical reproduction or translation reserved.

info@bircher-benner.com   www.bircher-benner.com
© Copyright by Edition Bircher-Benner, CH-8784 Braunwald
® The trademarks Bircher and Bircher-Benner are protected worldwide

The suggestions in this book have been carefully considered and reviewed by the authors and the publisher. Nevertheless, we cannot assume any guarantee. Liability of the authors or the publisher for injury or damage to property, personal or other, or financial loss are excluded.

Cover design: Kösel Media GmbH, Krugzell
Overall production: Kösel, Krugzell

Table of contents

Preface to the 32nd edition 7

Introduction 8

The structure and function of the liver 9
    The enterohepatic cycle as a vicious circle 12

The tasks of the liver 14

Scientific bases of the order therapy for liver-gallbladder disease 18
    The problem with small amounts of alcohol 21

The different disease forms of the liver-gallbladder system 24
    The general appearance of the failing liver function and first measures 24
    Inflammation of the liver (hepatitis) 25
    Liver cirrhosis (cirrhotic liver) 28
    Liver failure as the final stage of liver cirrhosis 29
    Tumour diseases of the liver 29
    Diseases of the gallbladder 30
    Gallbladder carcinoma 32
    Bile-duct stones (choledocholithiasis) 32
    Postcholecystectomy syndrome 32

Plant remedies for liver-gall diseases (phytotherapy, spagyrics) 34
    Treatment of infections 35

Hydrotherapy 37
    Compresses 37
    Gushes 38
    The baths 39
    Washes 40

Compresses and applications	41
Description of some water applications and compresses	42

Homeopathic therapy, miasmatically inherited consequences of diseases and traumas ... 44

The new scientific acupuncture ... 46

Neural therapy according to Huneke ... 47

Surgical Procedures ... 49

The healing plan	50
The healing regime	50
Treatment of hepatitis	51
Treatment of liver cirrhosis	52
Treatment of gallbladder inflammation (cholecystitis)	53
To prevent and avoid relapses	53
The four diet stages	56
Diet Stage I – The raw-juice regime	56
Diet Stage II	58
The Stage-III Diet	59
The Stage-IV Diet	62
Small substitution table for animal products that must be left out in the stage-III diet	63
The Recipes	64
Juices	64
Healthful Teas	65
Birchermuesli	66
Raw vegetables and Salads	68
Salad dressings	69
Milk Types	71
Butter, plant and vegetable fats and oils – Light cooking and steaming	72
Soups	73
Vegetables	76
Salads of cooked vegetables	81

Potato dishes	82
Cereal Dishes	85
Sauces	87
Sandwiches	89
Desserts	90
List of recipes	93
Bibliography	96
Glossary	101

Preface to the 32nd edition

This manual is based on long experience in the treatment of patients who have been healed by Bircher's order therapy. The earlier editions have been supplemented with many notes from basic research and the new results of clinical gastroenterological research, and the dietetic section has also been slightly revised without losing the high quality of Bircher's recipes. The manual gives the patient or person with a weakness of the liver the required knowledge and the indispensable practical instruction to enable him to stop progression of his disease and initiate continuous healing steps.

The book can be a valuable aid for the doctor practicing holistic treatment, helping him or her to provide patients with instructions for changing their lifestyles towards the order therapy.

Since its establishment by Dr med. Max Oscar Bircher-Benner, the order therapy for liver and gall diseases has been researched for more than one hundred years at the Bircher-Benner clinic and in private practices under careful observation of its healing effects. Throughout these years, the many thousands of desperate patients who recovered from their rapidly worsening diseases have been our best teachers. With a strong will to be healed, they successfully followed the instructions of the order therapy and enabled great insights whose confirmation is only now slowly being reflected in general medical research.

In the change to a more healthful lifestyle, nutrition is of primary importance! It leads to regeneration of the large regulation systems, a new opening towards the outer world and oneself that permits the healing forces of the organism, body and soul to begin their work. Let me finally quote a section of Bircher-Benner's book *Vom Werden des neuen Arztes (Genesis of the New Physician):* "The wonders of the soul remain closed to those who continually ignore the laws of nutrition. Power and depth of inner experiences depend on nutrition – this is their actual meaning. Taking care of one's body and nutrition is useless unless a new development and awakening of inner powers results from it."

Dr med. Andres A. Bircher

Introduction

In recent decades, the number of people suffering from liver diseases or their consequences or who are aware of having a "sensitive liver" has greatly increased (Li et al.).

Only part of this trend is due to epidemic liver inflammations (hepatitis), which often cause a permanent condition of oversensitivity to certain foods, flatulence and a general reduction of strength even after apparent healing. Additionally, however, liver function is stressed by general, wide-spread nutritional damage, alcohol, pharmaceutical poisons and a sedentary lifestyle causing lack of circulation in the liver due to shallow breathing and insufficient movement, as well as the permanent nervous tension of our times, all of which make recovery after damage considerably more difficult.

The liver patient is aware that the function of his liver is reflected in its adaptability to food. He knows that dietary mistakes have direct consequences. The consequences are not only local complaints in the area of the liver, such as flatulence, slow digestion, burping, tension and a heavy feeling, but also an irritating disturbance of the general feeling of life, of the freshness of life and the ability to perform, of mood and of relationships with other people. After a setback, one feels oppressed, irritable and defenceless, withdraws into oneself or inadvertently hurts others and is unable to do anything.

The liver patient generally observes which foods he has to avoid. He protects his liver as well as he can, His conclusions, his knowledge of the construction and function of the liver and his will are, however, not always adequate to prevent important mistakes in his lifestyle that prevent healing of his liver-gallbladder condition.

This little book is based not only on the latest scientific insights, but also on more than one hundred years of practical clinical experiences at the Bircher-Benner clinic. It will give the reader all the knowledge that he needs to make his own contribution to healing.

The dietetic section contains recipes and practical regimes that have been developed in close cooperation of the dietary kitchen with doctors from the Bircher-Benner clinic.

The recipes are appealing in their taste and variety. The liver-gallbladder diet thus can be enjoyed by the patient so that it is not experienced as a limitation, but as a exploratory journey into a new world, a healthy, pleasant new way of living and eating.

The structure and function of the liver

The liver holds a central position in the organism's metabolism. The metabolic performance of the biochemical "power plant" of every single cell in the body is reinforced many times over in the liver cell. Additionally, the organ has special metabolism, synthesis and storage functions. The liver, which accounts for only 3 % of the body's weight, performs 12 % of the total metabolic work. The fact that a liver cell has to work four times as hard as an average body cell shows how great the effect of functional impairment and disease of the liver may be on the health of the entire organism.

Functionally, the liver is connected to the lateral longitudinal thirds of the body with the periphery of the sympathetic nervous system. These are the lateral control systems of soft connective tissue, as well as the nerve and muscle chains that are used for all turning movements and for "making room to the side".

Traditional Chinese healing connects fulfilment, vitality, courage, elasticity, anger and hustle and bustle with total energy in the function cycle of the liver, but timidity, lack of courage and bitterness with weakness of the liver as "inner factors" or characteristics. According to the traditional Chinese approach, an excessive liver function often coincides with painful inflammation of the tendons and excessive muscle movement, while liver weakness is reflected in a lack of muscle strength, paralysing weakness and inertia. In the German language, such experiences are also reflected in expressions like "vor Zorn läuft ihm die Galle über" ("his bile overflows in fury") or the term "bitterness", the taste that we find in bile and all cholagogic medication, as an expression of suppressed, restrained fury, the fury of "Rumpelstiltskin", who suppresses his inner fury until he tears himself apart.

These holistic Ancient Chinese and European folklore observations are confirmed in everyday medicine, as is the connection between functional impairment of the liver and the eyes, where surges of unrestrained energy may be expressed as itching, redness, inflammation or trigeminusneuralgia, and weakness may appear as visual problems.

The energetic-functional interrelation of the liver with headache and migraine is better known. Where the excessive function causes heat accumulation with explosive pounding pain, functional weakness is experienced as emptiness and drowsiness. Energy overflow and emptiness are conducted in the vascular bundles of the connective tissue (meridians) and the vegetative nerve fibres along the vessels. The anatomy of the meridians and acupuncture points has been determined (Heine, 1985, 1987).

All changes such as drafts and winds, changing weather, puberty and menopause are properties or stages of life that particularly stress the liver-gallbladder system according to traditional Chinese opinion. Thus we find that anxiety, agitation and sleeplessness, migraines, and sensitivity to drafts and weather occur increasingly during menopause, as do enervating hot flushes, which can be understood as unrestrainedly rising energy discharges from the function circle of the liver. Traditional Chinese opinion explains this unrestrainedness of liver energy by the reduction of the energy in the sexual organs, which are now no longer able to regulate the liver with their usually inhibiting effect.

Let us note there that all of these holistic Eastern observations are attributed to purely pragmatic medicine, which so far has only been partially proven by our current scientific method. But they are confirmed in the daily practice of a carefully observant doctor. The doctor on emergency standby will usually be called to his patients for gall colic in the earliest morning, just after midnight: according to Ancient Chinese opinion, the function circle of the liver-gallbladder system has its greatest energetic activity during that time.

Anatomically, the liver is made up of three lobes. The large right liver lobe in the right upper abdomen rests against the diaphragm dome and reaches far up into the thorax (see schematic illustration, p. 17). The left, much smaller liver lobe can be felt near the tip of the sternum just below the costal arch. Between these organ lobes, where the third, small, square liver lobe and the gallbladder are also located, large vessels and the bile ducts lead into the organ. Therefore, this location is also called the porta hepatis. Here, in a strong band that holds the liver, there are the closed residues of the umbilical vessels, which become permeable again in chronic portal vein congestion and are sometimes responsible for star-shaped venous expansions that become visible on the belly around the navel (Caput medusae).

The liver lobes are made up of an immense number of polyangular liver lobules that are barely recognisable with the unaided eye. They form a kind of functional units and give the liver its fine-grained look. Each of these liver lobules is supplied from a dedicated vessel and has its own lymphatic vessel and bile duct system (see schematic illustration, p. 17).

A dedicated artery trunk from the aorta strongly supplies the liver with oxygen-rich blood. The portal vein is a second large blood-supply system, a vascular trunk that collects all blood from the small intestine, the spleen and two-thirds of the large intestine and supplies it to the liver. This blood contains the food components and toxins to be excreted from the intestine and cell degradation products from the spleen, which serves to rejuvenate and clean the blood.

Where three of the honeycomb-like interlocked liver lobules meet, we will find the branches of the liver artery, the portal vein and the bile duct (ductus choledochus). From there, capillary nets from the artery and the portal vein weave around the liver lobules and rest against each individual liver cell in sequence, thus running into the very inside of the liver lobules, where they connect and empty their blood into the small central vein after intense substance and gas exchange. These hepatic veins in the middle of the many thousand liver lobules combine like many small brooks into a river and meet in the large hepatic vein, which finally empties all the blood from the liver into the large body vein (the vena cava). Each liver lobule also contains a finely built lymph-drainage system (tissue drainage) and is supplied by many vegetative nerve endings.

Every single liver cell is enveloped by the basic substance of the soft connective tissue (Pischinger, 1990). All vegetative nerve fibres end independently in this basic substance, which regulates the information and substance exchange of the liver in the manner of a molecular screen. Each substance and each piece of information that is to reach or leave the liver cell must go through this basic substance of the soft connective tissue. The quality of the basic substance is decisive for the regulation capacity and thus the health of the liver. It mostly depends on the quality of nutrition and cannot be regenerated by medication, but only by suitable healing foods (Eppinger et al. 1939).

The honey-thick yellow-green bile is formed in each liver cell and collected in the bile capillaries surrounding them. Following the course of the liver artery and portal vein, the branched bile ducts collect in a single large bile duct (ductus choledochus), that connects with the gallbladder at the porta hepatis. The gallbladder serves to thicken the bile continually formed by the liver and to keep it ready for the moment of the meal. This bile supply is a viscous, thread-forming, almost black mass called "B-bile". Only when a meal is eaten will the gallbladder reflexively empty itself into the discharging bile duct in several contractions, from there into the pancreatic duct (ductus pancreaticus) and together with the juice of the pancreas into the duodenum.

The gallbladder is a very important organ for substance excretion via the intestine. Its bile acids give stool its dark colour and also help split and digest fats and oils. The quality of bile – its content in the different bile acids and bile dyes – is decisive for the digestive function and health of the intestine. For example, patients suffering from carcinoma of the large intestine have a detrimental composition of bile acids. Types of bile acids have been found that irritate the rectum and thus contribute to the chronic rectum inflammation (proctitis) that precedes the cancer.

The function of the liver depends on good blood supply, which adjusts precisely to the working demand of the organ. It may be increased up to fourfold. Under certain circumstances, it may also act as a blood reserve for the organism, if the oxygen content of the blood in the liver artery drops because of circulation problems, e.g. cardiovascular disease, or insufficient breathing and movement of the body. The functioning of liver cells suffers considerably from a lack of supply with oxygen. This lack of oxygen in the liver has a fatal effect on the organ, causing a slow fatty degeneration that starts at the centre of the lobules. The liver loses its functional performance and liver stress tests show that its detoxification work is slowed down and bile production reduced.

Nutrition that is too rich in fat, free carbohydrates or protein puts too much of a stress on the liver after each meal with excess glucose and the organic acids arising from the degradation of excessive fats and amino acids. The excessive nutrients then act as nutritional toxins and massively increase the fatty degeneration of the liver.

In this over-strain of the liver during its metabolic and detoxification function, it has to pass on the acids that it cannot handle in terms of metabolic function to the bile or venous blood. If the inflowing acid flood after meals is so high that the alkaline reserves are not enough to maintain the acid-base balance, the entire body will store organic acids as waste products in the basic substance of the soft connective tissue. They impair its function as a molecular sieve, the information and substance conduction system that controls the substance, gas and information exchange of the body cells, particularly the liver cells. What was once the almost embryonically soft connective tissue of the liver thickens and hardens and fills with metabolic waste products. The fatty degeneration of the liver slowly turns into scarred degeneration: liver cirrhosis.

Metabolism is not the liver's task alone. The substance and information exchange of all cells in the body is controlled by the basic substance of the soft connective tissue. But the metabolic work not performed by the liver cannot be accomplished in the rest of the body. Organic acids and other metabolic residues collect in all tissues and thus cause the large degenerative diseases caused by the faulty nutrition now generally prevalent, such as arteriosclerosis and coronary sclerosis, heart attack, rheumatic diseases (cf. Bircher-Benner manual no. 10 "Manual for patients with rheumatism and arthritis"), certain skin conditions, osteoporosis, hormonal and metabolic problems and many other diseases. The risk of cancer is massively increased (Stehelin, 1993; Chang et al., 1992, 1993).

The enterohepatic cycle as a vicious circle

The liver, overstressed by oxygen deficit, poor nutrition and alcohol, tries to discharge much of the excessive inflow of substances through the bile. Thus the bile loses its healthy composition. Individual metabolic components are now excreted in it at such high concentration that they precipitate into the gallbladder, where the bile is thickened most, and form gall grit or gallstones.

Gallstones irritate the mucous membrane of the wall of the gallbladder and cause chronic gallbladder inflammation (cholecystitis). Gallbladder colic is well known, and is caused by a sudden congestion of the gallbladder duct or bile duct in its further course. The painful colic at the upper abdomen is massive and unbearable and requires immediate medical help. Congestion of the bile drain by the gallstones also causes a backlog of the bile into the liver. Caustic bile, damaging to tissue, floods the finely formed liver lobules and harms them. It can flow off only through the small central hepatic veins and thus enters the blood circulation and all tissues, causing jaundice (Verdinicterus), first visible at the white of the eye, then also in the skin. We will deal with this condition again later.

Even if there is no bile accumulation, the other unhandled metabolic waste products of the bile will enter the small intestine through the bile ducts, irritate the intestinal mucous membrane with their toxic effect and noticeably impair the microbial environment, the intestinal flora. The intestine is irritated, is overgrown with putrefying pathogens, and becomes sensitive, flatulent and ill. The mucous membrane loses its ability to reject allergens. Various food components, usually first milk proteins and wheat constituents, are no longer compatible and *increase* the irritation. Putrefaction products and inflammation substances from the intestinal environment are added to the toxins swamping the intestine from the overstressed liver. All of this in turn is returned to the liver by the intestine through the portal vein for detoxification. This vicious circle between the damaged intestine and the over-stressed liver is closed and becomes a single, larger interference field for the entire organism. Bloating, fallen bowels, adiposity of the belly, impaired stool emptying, haemorrhoids and metabolic disorders of the cholesterol, fat and uric-acid cycle are the consequence, contributing to the arteriosclerosis and rheumatic symptoms.

We can thus consider the cholesterol and uric-acid content of the blood an expression of this metabolic task long before they exceed the permitted standard limits. Cholesterol and uric-acid levels are valuable parameters that show the patient and the attending physician whether the nutrition change has been implemented successfully and consistently enough.

Haemorrhoids also provide an indication that the above-described enterohepatic cycle is overloaded. Natural healing considers bleeding haemorrhoids a kind of valve outlet, a sign that the enterohepatic cycle urgently needs to be relieved. Surgery is not required from that point of view. If the nutrition is changed correctly, they will usually heal entirely.

The tasks of the liver

The liver's functions are so diverse that we must be more amazed and full of admiration the more we deal with them. It is even suspected that not all its functions are entirely known yet. The liver doubtlessly is a central organ of life. Its location – in the upper part of the abdomen, along the diaphragm – causes it to push against the diaphragm when swollen, possibly impairing breathing and impinging on the heart. It may also put pressure on the stomach, the intestine, the bile ducts and the large abdominal vessels. Inflammation in the area around the porta hepatis (liver hilus), e.g. in the area of the gallbladder, the bile duct, the duodenum or the stomach, may spread from one organ to the other in the open duct system that connects them all. Therefore, doctors also call this area the "weather corner", because in healing the whole, the harmony in cooperation and dependence of all parts on each other must be kept in view. Otherwise, the intended final goal cannot be achieved. We will talk about this in detail below.

Let us now give you a brief overview of the tasks of the liver.

Secretion:
Bile production

Tasks in the metabolism:
1) Carbohydrate metabolism: transfer of the carbohydrates from the intestine into a consistent form (glycogen)
2) Protein metabolism: amino acid degradation, urea and uric acid metabolism
3) Fat metabolism: The excretion of bile permits splitting and resorption of fats from the intestine. The liver is able to convert excessive fats into sugars.
4) Mineral metabolism: regulation of the acid-base balance
5) Water metabolism: in connection with the hormonal glands and the kidneys
6) Heat balance, heat generation
7) Vitamin synthesis (vitamins of the B-group, D, A, K)

Storage tasks:
1) Vitamin storage
2) Iron and copper storage (blood formation)
3) Storage of other factors for blood formation
4) Glycogen storage (glycogen, also called animal starch, is a storable form of carbohydrates)
5) Fat storage
6) Protein storage

Detoxification tasks:
Food toxins and bacteria toxins are disintegrated in the liver.

Regulation of the sensitivity and defence reactions to harmful food and environmental influences, destruction of germs in infections by viruses, bacteria and fungi, regeneration and repair of damaged tissues:
The liver is particularly rich in the connective tissue that specializes in this function, the defence cells that make up the so-called reticulo-endothelial system, which is spread throughout the body, but particularly in the bone marrow, the liver, the spleen and thymus.

At the embryonic stage, blood and immune-cell formation initially happens in the liver, spleen and thymus. Only just before birth will the bone marrow actually take over this task. The spleen specialises in the collection and degradation of old blood cells. The thymus behind the sternum is the organ of origin of lymphatic cell formation and thus of the immune system.

The reticulo-endothelial system includes all cells of the blood and immune system. Even though spread through the body, it always reacts as a whole. Therefore, damage to the liver always has an appreciable effect on blood formation and the immune system of the organism.

Task in blood coagulation:
1) Production of the coagulation factor fibrinogen
2) Production of the coagulation factor prothrombin
3) Production of the blood platelets

Regulation of the blood volume:
Blood storage

Hormonal task:
The liver interacts with the adrenal glands and the ovaries in a way that is still partially unexplained.

We shall now select a few more tasks from the many that can now be considered specifically.

The carbohydrate metabolism:
The liver stores sugar by connecting sugar molecules into chains (polymerisation), producing glycogen (animal starch).
The liver is able to convert excess food fats and proteins into sugar and store it as glycogen. The glycogen storage of the liver is vital for continuous availability of glucose; without it, the brain would die within three minutes. The function of the liver cells also vitally depends on this store.

If the glycogen store is insufficient, as happens in areas with famine, the organism will become susceptible to infection and is insufficiently protected from degeneration and poisoning.

The best glycogen sources are foods with sugars that are released slowly, such as fruit and uncooked wholegrain. The natural glucose forms liver glycogen much better than do industrial sugars or glucose without the vital substances. For top performance in short-duration sports, it is therefore advisable to ingest a fast-acting carbohydrate source just before starting. Dried fruit or honey would be better here than glucose.

Muscle work causes the liver to use up glycogen in order to provide it to the muscle cells as glucose. Thus the blood-sugar level is maintained by muscle work. If the liver loses its glycogen reserves, sugar regulation will be impaired. Undesired fluctuations of the blood-sugar level occur, leading to regulation problems in the vegetative nervous system and in the inner secretory glands (hormonal glands), the pituitary gland, the adrenal gland, the thyroid gland, the ovaries, etc. Blood-sugar stress curves therefore are very important for diagnosis of liver diseases. Impaired storage function of the liver may mimic diabetes.

The protein metabolism:
The liver builds body protein from the amino acid mixtures of the food proteins. Protein circulates in the blood as plasma albumin, the transport form of the body's protein. Its level is kept constant by the liver. All body cells get their own supply from the plasma albumin. Hunger causes the liver to emit its protein reserves. Only then will body tissue be broken down to maintain the protein level.

The same "self-digestion" of the body happens when the liver is sick and unable to build up protein anymore. The protein concentration in the blood then drops slowly. To help patients with this condition, one often tries to balance out the loss by nutrition rich in protein or to remove the deficit by infusion of plasma albumin. The first measure is hardly effective, the second effective only briefly.

The Bircher-Benner therapy suggests a different approach, which has now been used by a number of other clinics and doctors as well. It assumes that an inflammatory or degeneratively ill liver that is no longer able to handle its regular tasks mostly requires protection rather than increased stress to achieve its urgently needed regeneration.

To protect the liver, the amount of food is reduced and the protein content is kept low, limited to those protein types that stress the liver metabolism as little as possible.

This property is determined by the amino acid composition of the protein. One such protein is casein, which is best digestible in the form of lean quark, buttermilk or natural fresh yoghurt at a carefully chosen amount, together with vegetable protein of green leaves, potatoes and whole gain.

The casein protein of milk contains liver-protecting factors that prevent fattening and death of the liver cells. Meat and other concentrated protein would cause a much higher metabolism strain on the liver and thus are left out entirely, at least for the duration of treatment in the Bircher-Benner clinic. We often observe that liver patients who had not recovered when eating mostly meat suddenly improved under a lacto-vegetarian diet with enough fresh vegetable food. Using an approach similar to Bircher-Benner's, other clinics and doctors replaced the "protein-rich regime" with 130–200 g/day of carbohydrate-rich, low-fat food. These included the former Eppingerklinik in Vienna, the Heilmeier and Kalk clinics and the Badadrie Clinic in Canada, where the protein supply for acute hepatitis was reduced to 30 g per day.

However, it must not be forgotten that an excess of all other nutrients additionally stresses the liver. Therefore, the best metabolic performance of the diseased liver is achieved by performance economy, i.e. with food that offers the liver no excess nutrients, but only what the organism absolutely needs at any given time.

All in all, it can be said that 50–70 g protein per day is already sufficient and that the protein supply for acute liver diseases may be reduced to 40–25 g/day to protect the liver with suitable selection of foods as described above. In acute cases, fat should be avoided entirely and the fructose supply should come mostly from fresh fruit, fresh vegetables and honey.

The extremely starved persons after World War II did not – as initially assumed – show only protein deficit, but a deficit of all nutrients, with the lack of trace elements, vital substances, minerals and carbohydrates causing liver failure and therefore danger to life.

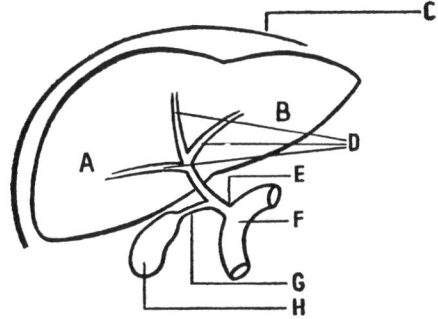

Schematic diagram of the liver, gallbladder and bile ducts

A = right liver lobe
B = left liver lobe
C = diaphragm
D = collecting ducts for liver-bile
E = large bile duct
F = duodenum
G = gallbladder duct
H = gallbladder

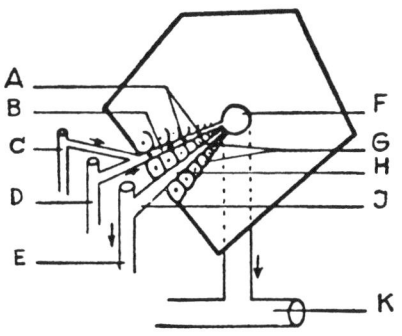

Schematic of a liver lobule according to Movill

A = Kupffer's cell
B = blood capillaries
C = branch of the liver artery
D = branch of the portal vein
E = bile duct
F = central vein
G = liver cells
H = small bile duct
I = Hernig's duct
K = branch of the vein

Scientific bases of the order therapy for liver-gallbladder disease

Lab examinations at our clinic (Liechti-v. Brasch et al., 1956; Kunz, 1948) document that the serum albumin level usually does not drop any further under our diet, but increases slowly. The food amount in general was kept low – the protein content was at 30–50 g/day. The composition of the amino acids was adjusted as precisely to demand as possible. The diet was low in fat and rich in raw fresh vegetable food. The progress of the serum albumin during treatment ensures that the body does not lose more protein, but that liver function recovers (Bircher-Benner, 1937; Kunz, 1948; Liechti-v. Brasch and Kunz, 1956; Liehti-v. Brasch, 1970; 1979).

Bohn and Runge (1938) confirmed the positive effect of raw-food therapy in liver cirrhosis and ascites (liquid collections in the abdominal space) in 1938. They recommended fresh vegetable juices for prophylaxis, also after recently cured acute liver diseases (hepatitis), which according to experience may turn into liver cirrhosis. Bircher's experience also confirmed that the raw-food therapy greatly facilitates alcohol abstinence, which is so decisive for liver patients (Kollenbach, 1974).

Friedrich and Peters (1939) report convincing therapy success with this treatment for the most severe forms of liver cirrhosis. They speak of a "downright life-saving effect of a raw-food therapy started in the most dangerous moment at the worst prognosis". To explain the good fresh-food effect, they refer to examinations of Eppinger (1938, 1939) and Kaunitz (1936) on the transmineralisation effect of raw food, and of Noorden (1929), who classified raw food as an antiphlogistic (antiinflammatory) therapy. Corresponding with Bircher-Benner, Friedrich and Peters (1939) supplemented the raw-food therapy for liver diseases with physical measures and focal restoration (removal of foci, interferences in the organism). Like Eppinger, Bohn and Runge, they prophylactically demanded the same treatment approaches for acute liver parenchyma diseases (diseases of the liver cells, such as hepatitis) (Kollenbach, 1974).

With the knowledge of the molecular-biological basics regarding storage of excess nutrients in the basic substance of the soft connective tissue and thus the relocation of the transit route between the cells and their surrounding structures (Pischinger, 1990), we can understand that adiposity means a massive nutrition and metabolism impairment of the tissues and the liver. The adipose person is actually in a constant condition of hunger, a vicious circle in which he eats because he is hungry, but causes the precise opposite: further stress on the liver and clogging of the basic substance with even worse cellular metabolism deficits. After all, he not only eats too much but particularly the wrong things. It has become clear that adiposity can be treated sustainably and successfully not by calorie reduction, but by raw juice treatment and subsequent raw-food therapy for nine months at free food volume (Bircher-Benner, 1933, 1938).

In the vicious circle of adiposity, intestinal symbiosis (the impaired intestinal flora) with the connected weakening of the liver and the enterohepatic cycle is also important (Bircher-Benner, 1933, 1938). There is little being done in adiposity research at the moment. Wadden et al. achieved at least a 10 % sustainable weight reduction with their partially order-therapeutic treatment and a supporting change of "lifestyle", and observe a significant improvement of the blood pressure values and serum cholesterol. Astrup et al. reported in 1990 that fibre addition to a hypocalorific common diet alone removed the cravings and constipation.

The liver is the key organ for regulating the fat and cholesterol levels in the blood. These levels express the metabolisms of the liver. There are many studies on reduction of the cholesterol level by dietetic measures (Barlow et al., 1990; Watts et al., 1992 and many others). They are of great interest to the medical profession because of the heart-attack risk. In 1988, the NCEP (National Cholesterol Education Program) was published in the USA, after many studies had documented the advantage of lipid reduction against heart-attack risk. Results from the great "Coronary Primary Prevention Trial" had asserted the famous 2:1 relation, according to which a cholesterol reduction by 1 % reduces the coronary heart-disease risk by 2 %. The dietary provisions of the AHA (American Heart Association) have been adjusted to these studies (Bae, 1991). The Helsinki heart study then showed that additional increase of the HDL (High-density lipoprotein) cholesterol values improves this result. Fibres such as bran or psyllium seeds have also been shown to reduce lipids several times (White, 1992; Keenan et al., 1991; Cara et al., 1991; Bell et al., 1990; Neal et al., 1990; Levin et al., 1990 and others).

A positive effect of unsaturated fatty acids (Omega-3-fatty acids) has been documented several times (Skuladottir et al., 1990 and many others). Gans et al. (1990) were able to show that Omega-3-fatty acids improved blood viscosity by helping the red blood cells regain their flexibility. Nephrosis (protein loss in the urine by basal-membrane damage at the kidney capillary loops) leads to considerable increase of blood fats as an expression of the regulation impairment of the entire liver metabolism. D'Amico et al. (1991) were able to show that the serum cholesterol levels in these patients will drop after drastic protein reduction in the diet.

When looking at these individual effects as a whole, all of them indicate a vegetable diet. There is a large number of papers that document that vegetable nutrition with a strong reduction of animal products is most effective in reducing lipids (three works of Singh et al., 1992, a,b,c; Yinnon et al., 1992; Sciarrone et al., 1992; Bernard, 1991 et. al.). Melchert et al. (1987, veget. Study 5) examined the differences of the entire lipid status in 62 female and 40 male vegetarians, and compared them to that of an omnivorous control group. Unsaturated oleic acids in particular were taken up moreby the vegetarians. The fatty acid composition of the cholesterol esters, triglycerides, free fatty acids and phosphatidylcholin was analysed. In all of these fractions, the fatty acid profile reflected the dietetic lipid intake. Palmitol, vaccenyl and docosahexoaenyl acid remained much lower in the serum of vegetarians. The greatest difference was measured for linoleic acid in all lipid classes, particularly in di- and triglycerides.

Where these insights, new at the time, were used consistently for therapy, they had a drastic effect on the risk of dying from coronary heart disease by improving the liver metabolism: A drastic reduction of LDL-cholesterol and overall cholesterol in the diet reduced the cases of coronary heart disease by 35 % and the need for surgical intervention in the coronary vessels by ⅔. The "Coronary Drug Project" and the "Multiple Risk Factor Intervention Trial", two large-scale prospective studies, documented the long-term effect of lipid reduction. Two other large studies proved the effect of dietetic lipid reduction angiographically as well (CLAS: cholesterol-Lowering Atherosclerosis Study and FATS: Familial Atherosclerosis Treatment Study). The FATS study additionally showed that an already-present arteriosclerosis of the coronary arteries can partially remit under a consistent lipid-reducing diet (cf. summary: Gotto, 1991). In all of these positive results, it must be considered that a drastic lipid reduction is only possible by very strong limitation of animal food, so that studies cannot only refer to cholesterol. Wood et al. (1991) showed that the effect of dietetic lipid reduction on coronary heart risk can be clearly improved by regular physical training in overweight men and women.

A breakthrough was achieved by Ornish et al. (1990) at the University of San Francisco with the randomised controlled study on the influence of nutrition and "lifestyle" on coronary sclerosis. During one year, 28 patients with advanced coronary sclerosis were at least partially treated order-therapeutically. They ate purely vegetarian with a very low share of saturated fats and did not smoke. They also received a certain relaxation training and instructions for adjusted physical training. Lipid reducing medication was not given. The control group comprised 20 patients precisely comparable in age, gender and coronary angiography findings (narrowing of the vascular cross-section by 40 %). The control group was treated according to all common recommendations of the American Heart Association. After one year, another angiography was performed. The order therapy group showed a clear reduction of complaints and expansion of the vessel cross-section from 40 % to 37.8 % narrowing (reduction of constriction), while the control group had suffered further constriction, on average from 42.7 to 46.1 % and clear increase of the complaints.

This outstanding work impressively demonstrates the great importance of nutrition for the liver metabolism and thus the blood lipid profile and its direct important influence on arteriosclerosis. It bears out the decades-long experience of the Bircher-Benner clinic, according to which a suitable change of diet will clear the tissues and permit already-narrowed vessels to open again. Dougall et al. also reported on the quick reduction of the cholesterol level from a low-fat, strictly vegetarian regime in 1995.

Fatty degeneration (fatty liver) is often connected to general overweight (metabolic syndrome). Adventist youths (vegetarians) are much less adipose than omnivorous comparison groups (Ritter et al., 1995). Vegetarians have only half the mortality risk for any food-dependent chronic diseases and in particular cancer and cardiovascular diseases (Chang et al., 1992 and 1993). This was already proven in Berlin in 1990 (Rottka, 1990).

The fatty liver can be improved by alcohol abstinence with weight reduction and physical training (Rich, 1996; Park et al., 1995; Ueno et al., 1997). With a suitable diet, even fast weight reduction of adipose patients with a fatty liver will not cause gallstones (Heshka et al., 1996). Fatty liver often occurs in celiac disease (malabsorption with food allergy) (Christi et al., 1999; Zippelius et al., 1999). These papers clearly demonstrate toxic stress of the liver due to excessive stress on the enterohepatic cycle (poisoning of the liver by toxins from the intestine).

The risk for developing gallstones increases with higher body weight (Zapata et al., 2000), which causes inertia of the gallbladder. Portincasa et al. (2000) find a more inert gallbladder in persons suffering from gallstones as well. The same applies after stomach surgery (Hahm et al., 2000). In a large-scale examination in New Delhi, Tandon et al. (1996) found that all gallstone patients had a much increased share of carbohydrates and the men also of saturated fats in their food. The triglyceride levels in the blood were strongly increased in all gallstone patients.

The bile of adipose persons contains cholesterol crystals. The slower the passage through the large intestine, the more likely are gallstones, which are attributable to changed bile-acid resorption (Thomas et al., 2000). Children with wrong nutrition also suffer from gallstones, which will disappear again under a suitable regime (Bruch et al., 2000). Tseng et al. (2000) showed that Mexican men had only half the risk of developing gallstones with a high proportion of vegetable food in their diets. High insulin levels, such as result from the consumption of much sugar and white flour, increase the gallstone risk (Ruhl et al., 2000). A sitting lifestyle and nutrition rich in animal fats, sugar and white flour, while also being low in fruit, vegetables and vegetable oils, causes gallstones much more often (Misciagna et al.,1999; Everhart, 1998; Caroli et al., 1998; Attili et al., 1998). Socha et al. (1998) showed that the content of unsaturated vegetable oleic acids has an essential influence on the bile flow in children with cholestasis. When diet fasting, adipose people only develop gallstones if the calorie-reduced diet contains saturated fats (Festi et al., 1998). Vezina et al. (1998) showed, among others, that the fat content of the diet is not always the only risk factor for gallstones during dietary fasting.

Nutrition recommendations for liver cirrhosis and chronic hepatitis have remained contradictoryin the medical field: Corrao et al. (1995) suspect that a high lipid and low protein and carbohydrate share in the diet and alcohol have a very detrimental effect on progress. Other authors recommend a higher protein supply (Nielsen et al., 1995). A "fattening diet" is without effect in cirrhosis patients (Campillo et al., 1997). Other authors recommend addition of branched chain amino acids (Watanabe et al., 1996). All in all, there is therapeutic uncertainty, except for the option of indication for a liver transplant, which may be successful in children as well (Shephard, 1996).

The risk of developing a carcinoma of the gallbladder or bile ducts is much higher if one's diet is rich in sugar, with the mono and disaccharides being most detrimental. But vegetables and fruit – epidemiologically speaking – are protection factors (Moerman et al., 1995). Furthermore, fibre substances in the food also improve the glucose metabolism of the liver (Laurent et al., 1995).

The problem with small amounts of alcohol

The harm of "small" daily amounts of alcohol is currently disputed. Studies have shown that people with low wine consumption (approx. 2 small glasses of wine/day = approx. 30 g pure alcohol/day) are a little less likely to die of the consequences of coronary heart disease than abstinent persons and persons drinking more alcohol. The vast publicity of this result is understandable, since it supports daily habit. Wine-growing areas in particular saw a general recommendation from many doctors to their patients. In countries such as France, where wine is drunk regularly, the connection between coronary heart disease and blood fats (cholesterol) can be documented much less clearly. This is called the "French paradox". Even relatively low amounts of alcohol (42 g pure alcohol/day) considerably increase the cholesterol level, however (Gupta et al., 1994).

Never forget that people who drink "a little" wine with a meal usually take in much more than 30 ml pure alcohol/day. Important interpretation problems occurred in an Italian study (Attili et al., 1998).

Tsugare et al. (1992) showed that background characteristics of the "moderate drinkers", such as smoking, nutrition, etc., were much better than those of the abstinent persons and those who consumed more alcohol in a Japanese epidemiological prospective study across 7 years.

In a carefully considered editorial in the *Journal of the American Medical Association*, the problem is dealt with in more detail (Gisling, 1994). A table lists all persons who are harmed even by the smallest amounts of alcohol: people with alcohol problems among their blood relations (family risk of alcoholism), pregnant women and people suffering from diseases of the liver, the pancreas, weakness of the heart, too-high blood triglyceride values, degenerative nervous diseases and certain blood diseases. Even the "smallest amounts" are considered harmful here, and even the smallest amounts of alcohol should be completely avoided before work or driving. In fact, increased accident risk with machines and vehicles and reduced mental performance after the consumption of small amounts of alcohol have been documented in many cases (editorial article *Lancet*, 1973; Whitby et al., 1994; Waagh et al., 1989; Parker et al., 1974; Voytechovsky et al., 1970). Remembering that nowadays people drive cars or operate machines virtually every day, the recommendation of "small amounts of alcohol" becomes very problematic.

In 1992 Wannametzee et al. from the Royal Free Hospital in London documented in a large number of patients that persons suffering from angina pectoris are much more likely to die of sudden heart failure than abstinent persons if they drink even very small amounts of alcohol.

Alcohol leads to oxygen deficit in the liver cells, which will promote fatty degeneration of the liver lobules even at a low daily amount (Sherman et al., 1994). In rats, regular small amounts of alcohol caused a bile reflux into the pancreas and pancreatitis (Jalovara, 1988). Simsek et al. (1990) found fatty substance deposits in the pancreas in similar experiments, as well as detrimentally changed blood-fat values. Similar metabolism changes were documented in humans many times in the last 25 years (Webster, Baum et al., 1975 and many more).

The increased risk for some cancer types from alcohol consumption has also often been documented. It is partially connected to the weakening effect of alcohol on the cellular immune system. The increased risk for stomach ulcers, sleep disorders, emphysema of the lung and many other diseases cannot be dealt with in more detail here.

Gallstones are more common in alcohol-drinking persons than in abstinent ones (Tseng et al., 2000; Jayanthi et al., 1998; Attili et al.; 1998).

In larger amounts, alcohol is known to often cause a toxic liver inflammation. The prognosis is particularly severe, since the condition usually causes fibrosis, i.e. liver cirrhosis, quickly (Cabré et al., 2000). Persons with higher alcohol consumption also develop hepatitis C more often than abstinent persons (Lieber, 2000).

We can see that the research on the influence of food on liver-gallbladder diseases is in progress, though an actual breakthrough of insights, such as has occurred for coronary sclerosis, has not yet been achieved. At the moment, there is much more being done in researching the nutritional causes of cancer.

The different disease forms of the liver-gallbladder system

The general appearance of the failing liver function and first measures

A patient with several acute liver diseases always requires strict medical supervision or even care in a hospital. Therefore, the description of this disease does not belong in the scope of this little book. Even milder chronic conditions require careful medical examination and consulting, but the patient can considerably speed up his healing with the suggestions from this book.

A healthy liver is not felt. It works as a matter of course without being noticed.

A diseased liver is different. A dull pressure and feeling of bloating in the right upper abdomen occurs. The patient knows that he is tired for a while after eating. He feels unable to make an effort. He moves carefully because of this bloated feeling and often does not like to lie on the right side or the belly. He also knows that he is "sensitive" to certain foods and that he must only ingest them in very small amounts or must leave them out altogether. If he takes in a little more, e.g. at a party or dinner out, there will be unpleasant consequences: severe flatulence precedes chronic, stubborn constipation and reoccurs after each meal. The constipation is often followed by sudden, episodic diarrhoea, usually with intestinal cramps and lots of gas. The patient often feels a swelling of the liver and pain that seems to occur in wave-like episodes through the organ, remaining for a longer time at the lower edge, near the gallbladder. At the same time, he feels a lack of appetite, is disgusted with food, and experiences nausea for one or several days. The tongue is coated and shows changes particularly at the lateral edges. The white in the corner of the eye often shows typical yellow discoloration. Even at regular bilirubin values, the skin may be slightly yellowed, and there may be an unpleasant itch (true jaundice is described later).

The head feels heavy, dull and painful in the forehead and the neck when the patient awakens, and often also towards evening. Waking up in the morning often becomes a difficult fight. The eyelids appear swollen, hands and feet thick and stiff, and the wrists and ankles, and particularly the calf muscles, often ache. The morning urine is dark and concentrated. In the course of the morning, with increasing freshness of the body, it becomes watery clear and flows in large amounts (this is very typical for regulation impairment of the mineral and water metabolism due to liver damage). Towards evening, the liver patient becomes increasingly fresh. He often even enters a kind of nervous irritation that will not let him sleep and makes his thoughts circle quickly but with little result, instead of experiencing stillness, relaxation and true sleep. Creative persons can work best in this condition of being awake at night, while others try to distract themselves to "not waste time by sleeping". The night often becomes their day. This reversal severely stresses their metabolism, whose regulation is aligned with the circadian rhythm, with hormone releases adjusted to the course of the sun. Thus the ring of the vicious circle is closed.

On the worst days, the "attacks" will cause the patient to eat little because of a lack of appetite. Instinctively, he will seek out herbal teas, fruit juices, dry bread, gruel soup or cereal dishes, all without fat, until he slowly recovers a little and new stress causes the next relapse.

We should mention a warning sign that may be described too rarely and that we recommend that all patients with weak livers observe. A few days before a relapse, i.e. failure of the liver, the self-control, or healthy instinct, seems to be lost. Probably because of change of the secretion in the stomach and intestine, the patient craves foods that stress the liver (cf. unrestrained cravings during pregnancy). There is a sudden craving for chocolate or fatty, strongly spiced foods, fat cheese, bacon or fried food. If the patient gives in to such paradoxical cravings, relapse is certain; if he recognises the situation and acts with self-control, he will have won and his liver will thank him for it! A fasting day with peppermint tea, fruit juice or fruit (particularly grapefruit, berries, apples, ripe oranges) and some crisp bread with honey (no butter) may avert the danger. Sips of a little bitter tea during the day to stimulate bile flow, application of hot compresses on the liver after each meal and early bed rest after a heating bath (not overheating, just to stimulate blood flow), followed by a Priessnitz compress (see page 37), will hold back the incipient swelling. It will always pay off to proceed so drastically, since it prevents ten days of feeling ill.

Intestinal regulation must be observed strictly. It is best to start a resting and fasting day with a thorough emptying of the intestine by an enema (2–3 times one litre of chamomile tea). This practice detoxifies the lower parts of the large intestine and relieves the enterohepatic circulation. Then drink 1–2 glasses of Karlsbad spring water on an empty stomach in the morning for 1 to 2 weeks. Other natural measures for stimulating the intestine can be found in the chapter "The healing plan".

If such relapses occur over years, there will certainly be severe damage, and if control of the diet and lifestyle is not energetically pursued, all artificial aids or treatments will be in vain. The condition will progress to emaciation, colitis (inflammation of the large intestine), possibly migraine, gallstones, gallbladder inflammation with true gall colics and wave-like jaundice conditions. Now the whole personality and mood changes: the ability to be happy, inner security and trust are lost. An entire family's life can be overshadowed by this condition, since lack of drive, lack of initiative, distrust, depression, defeatism and underlying anger are the greatest enemies of a harmonious atmosphere in families and groups of people. Liver disease continued over many years will end in the risk of acute liver failure.

The described symptoms are just what we find in chronic liver diseases, such as chronic hepatitis or fatty liver, caused by wrong and excessive food or chronic poisoning, e.g. regular alcohol consumption or medication or the effect of toxins at work, etc.

Liver failure occurs when the liver no longer has enough functional liver lobules to make the vital metabolism work. All chronic liver diseases threaten to end like this in the form of liver cirrhosis, i.e. changing of the liver into an connective-tissue-like scarred condition.

Inflammation of the liver (hepatitis)

This is often just called "jaundice", although yellow skin colour occurs from any backlog of bile into the liver.

We differentiate between:

Infectious hepatitis
This usually is a viral infection. Exceptions are infections by parasites (malaria, tapeworms), yellow fever, leptospirosis or liver abscesses.

Viral hepatitis

Hepatitis A
This is also called "HA", "epidemic" or "infectious hepatitis". The germ is a 27 nm large ribonucleic-acid- containing picornavirus. Many infections happen unnoticed, often in childhood: the virus is ingested from fecal matter in contaminated foods or drinking water, so that this "jaundice" occurs in epidemics. The incubation time (time from infection to appearance of the disease) usually is 20–30 days. Stool and blood of the patient are infectious to others from the 2nd to the 6th week after infection.

The signs before the disease breaks out (prodromi) are continuous fatigue, exhaustion, lack of drive, usually depression, noticeably stubborn lack of appetite with sudden unmotivated cravings, often unusual, severe constipation, pressure in the heart, drowsiness, dizziness, fainting due to a drop in blood pressure. Then the disease breaks out with fever and strong general feeling of illness, often together with catarrhs; slight to severe jaundice usually develops in the course of a few days. First the eyes turn yellow, then the skin. An annoying itch announces the irritating effect of the bile acids in the blood serum. With incipient jaundice (icterus), the fever drops and the condition improves. Liver, spleen and lymph nodes swell, and the liver is painful. Stool turns light, pale, urine dark. In severe cases, there is a tendency to faint or even toxic continuous sleep.

Hepatitis A never enters a chronic stage and has the best prognosis of all liver inflammations. Antibodies remain in the blood for the life of the patient and reliably protect against reinfection.

Hepatitis B
"This is called "HB" or "serum hepatitis". The 42 nm large virus contains deoxyribonucleic acid and a hull that can be documented in the immune response of the organism as a surface antigen in the lab test. This is also called "Australia-Antigen" (HbsAG). The HbeAG (envelope) is another surface antigen and the HbcAG (core) the core antigen of the virus. These antigens are used in the lab test to document the virus, i.e. to determine if a person carries hepatitis B viruses and must take care not to infect others.

Infection takes place via the blood, i.e. when drawing blood, because of injury and blood contact or when drug addicts share needles.

The infection may also take place via contact with bodily excretions or during sexual intercourse. Therefore, persons in the medical professions, children of mothers positive for hepatitis (40 %), dialysis patients, haemophiliacs, drug addicts and persons in homosexual relationships are particularly endangered. Infection does not always occur from contact with the virus and is confirmed by the antibody proof (Anti HBs).

The incubation time is usually 50–90 days. The patient is contagious while the IgE antigen can be documented in the blood.

The symptoms are as described for hepatitis A. The jaundice continues for 1–4 weeks. In 90 % of cases, the disease heals fully. One out of every two hundred patients dies of acute destruction of the liver. Nearly every tenth develops chronic hepatitis B with the risk of development into cirrhosis (connective-tissue-like destruction and scarring of the liver).

Hepatitis C
This virus is most often transmitted in blood transfusions. The incubation time is 1–5 months. This disease progresses more or less like hepatitis B.

Hepatitis D
This is a virus that can only cause illness after hepatitis B and that will have a detrimental effect on its prognosis.

Hepatitis E
This Virus is found in epidemic liver inflammations in India, Africa, Asia and Central America. Its transfer and epidemiology correspond roughly to those of hepatitis A.

It is interesting that the hepatitis viruses can never harm liver cells directly (Harrisons, 1995). Some authors believe that cells are damaged by the immune response of the organism. Experiments by Mikhailova (1986) showed, however, that hepatitis can be transmitted directly through quartz glass without any effect of the virus, but only through UV-light-permeable quartz glass. This Russian researcher was able to prove that the transmission takes place by photon light spectrums in the UV range rather than by the virus. Scientists are still facing some fascinating questions here.

The general treatment of hepatitis is described in the chapter "The healing plan".

Therapy of hepatitis with medication
The history of medication for this disease is characterised by many apparent successes that turned out to be failures in the end. The high diagnostic differentiation of modern medicine is counterbalanced by a lack of clinical effectiveness and massive side effects.

At the moment, medicine gives interferon a the best chance. It is used for chronic hepatitis B, if the signs for virus reproduction are strong. Prospectively controlled studies have shown that patients with well-compensated chronically replicative hepatitis B reacted to antiviral therapy with interferon (Harrison, 1995).
A monthly injection for 4 months led to a certain reduction of the virus production in these patients and made the virus drop below the evidence threshold in about every tenth patient. The liver biopsy improved as well. Relapses after this are rare at 1–2 %. However, the success is clouded by very strong and partially very dangerous side effects that will not all disappear if the medication is discontinued. Use of interferon must be considered very carefully from case to case.

There are protective vaccinations against hepatitis A and B. Their use is disputed and should be critically considered in any case.

Other forms of infectious hepatitis
The mononucleosis caused by the Epstein-Barr virus, a viral disease of the entire organism, also affects the liver. In the acute stage, there is high fever, swelling of the liver and spleen, and inflammation of the tonsils. This condition is also called glandular fever. The virus remains in the body after healing, and the disease may continue at a low level and weaken the organism and the liver considerably. Under stress, the infection will easily be reactivated with a feeling of flu, great weakness and liver symptoms. Immune-strengthening therapy (see under therapy for infections) must be combined with the described general liver therapy.

Infections from *Echinococcus* (tapeworms), *Brucella*, toxoplasmosis, tropical diseases, etc. are rarer here and cannot be discussed in the scope of this book.

Toxic and medication hepatitis
There are 37 substance classes of medications that may cause partially dangerous

damage to the liver. Therefore careful discussion of possible side effects with the doctor and careful reading of the packaging leaflet before taking medication is important. During hepatitis, medication that is broken down in the liver or that has side effects on the liver must be discontinued if at all possible.

The best-known liver cell toxin is alcohol. Alcohol causes toxic hepatitis with a very bad prognosis, since it turns to liver cirrhosis even more often than does viral hepatitis. Its therapy is as for hepatitis.

In autumn, mushroom pickers are at risk of amanita poisoning. This toxic mushroom is very similar to the champignon. Poisoning will have devastating effects. It usually leads to acute destruction of the liver and death. Additionally there are occupational and environmental poisons that cannot be dealt with here.

Liver cirrhosis (cirrhotic liver)

As described above, the cirrhotic liver develops from the fatty liver, by further poisoning and degeneration, i.e. due to many years of harmful effects on the liver tissue and inflammations that never get to heal entirely. This includes scarring and shrinking of the entire liver, with increasing loss of functional liver lobules.

Causes include tropical diseases, poisoning, chronic alcohol use, certain sexually transmitted diseases, liver inflammations, rare congenital metabolism disorders of the liver (storage diseases), or simply diverse overload of the liver due to wrong and excessive food intake.

In the progressive stage, the cirrhotic liver becomes an obstacle to blood drain from the intestine, since the many small portal vein branches that are to take the blood from the intestine to the liver lobules are considerably reduced. There is an accumulation and pressure increase in the portal vein system. This blood accumulation in the intestine causes haemorrhoids, since the veins of the rectum are short-circuit connections between the portal vein and the hollow vein system that bypasses the liver circulation. These short-circuit connections in the form of the rectal veins swell into painful and often bleeding vein nodes, the haemorrhoids. Of course, the problem is not removed by haemorrhoid surgery, which only suppresses the valve effect and bleeding tendency.

A second such short-circuit connection bypassing the liver is the veins of the oesophagus. They, too, swell and may cause dangerous bleeding (bleeding oesophageal varices). The accumulation in the portal vein system finally causes water excretion into the abdominal cavity (ascites). The bile flow is impaired by the scarring of the liver and there will be jaundice (accumulation icterus).

Liver cirrhosis is a severe situation. The little liver tissue that still remains functional must be protected to the utmost and requires a careful diet, of course. Any mistake must be avoided. Warming the liver is important. Slight stimulation for bile formation by carefully chosen bitter teas, appropriate mineral waters and healing herbs is important, as well as strict intestinal regulation, as described in the chapter "The healing plan".

The mineral balance, impaired by the water loss, must be recovered by a careful raw food regime and lots of vegetable broth. The diet plan corresponds to the fat-free bland diet – with individual adjustment (see diet stage II).

Liver failure as the final stage of liver cirrhosis

When the connective-tissue-like scarring and shrinkage of the liver have progressed very far, there will be two symptoms that cause potentially fatal conditions. In the first place, the number of remaining functional liver lobules is no longer sufficient to detoxify even minimally the toxins supplied from the intestine through the portal vein.

The second phenomenon is the effect of the bypass circulations through the oesophageal vein, the re-opening umbilical vessels and the rectal veins (haemorrhoidal veins), since the cirrhotic liver massively impairs draining of the blood from the portal vein system in the small portal veins within the liver (portal vein hypertension due to drain impairment). The strongly toxin-containing blood from the intestine, which is also diseased, thus mostly does not return to the remaining liver lobules at all, but goes right into the main body circulation, and thus to the tissues of all organs. This effect may cause potentially fatal kidney failure (hepatorenal syndrome) or *hepatic encephalopathy*.

This is a toxin-related mental and mood disorder with strangely flapping tremor of the hands and the great danger of unconsciousness and death. Even in these life-threatening final conditions, strict monitoring and in-patient treatment consisting of intestinal detoxification by way of purely vegan fresh food therapy, initially administered only as fresh juices, can often have a life-saving effect.

Another complication of liver cirrhosis to be observed is the tendency to bleed, since the liver can no longer produce blood coagulants. This complication is reflected in flea-bite-like red haemorrhages of the skin, spontaneously appearing blue haemorrhages of the skin or bleeding from internal organs.

Tumour diseases of the liver

The most common benign *liver tumour* is the liver haemangioma, an always-benign vascular tumour that will be found in the ultrasound scan of one out of two hundred persons. It does not require any therapy.

Benign gland nodules of the liver (*liver adenomas*) have become very common in women since oral contraceptives have become popular. They can grow up to 10 cm. They must be diagnostically differentiated from malign tumours and may turn malign in about 10 % of cases. Therefore, they must be removed surgically if possible. They may also turn painful if they bleed or partially die.

Other benign tumours (*focal nodular hyperplasia*) are independent of contraceptives and do not turn malign, so that they can be left in place if they cause no problems. These are the most common benign tumours.

Liver carcinoma is a very malign tumour consisting of degenerated liver cells. In parts of Asia and Africa, 5 out of 1000 people develop this cancer ever year. In Europe and the USA, it is found in about every hundredth person who died of cancer. This type of cancer grows on the base of liver cirrhosis in 75 % of all cases. Hepatitis B plays a great role as another risk factor, since the risk is 100 times higher in persons infected with this virus.

In Europe and the USA, however, alcohol and faulty nutrition create the basis for this tumour, which can kill within 3 to 6 months. Surgical removal, if possible at all, will only extend life a little.

Otherwise, there is fibro-lamellar carcinoma, which appears independently of liver cirrhosis and in much younger persons. It grows much more slowly and has a five-year healing chance of 50 %.

Liver metastases most frequently result from primary tumours in the gastrointestinal tract, the lung, the female breast and from melanoma (pigment cells in the skin). Surgical measures or chemotherapy have only a slight life-extending effect, if any.

The chapter on scientific bases clearly shows the great importance of a diet in keeping with ours. The effectiveness of such nutrition has been amply documented for nearly all cancer types so far. Once the disaster has occurred, immune-strengthening "inner cancer therapy" often can have surprising effects. Unfortunately, we cannot deal with this matter in this scope of this book.

Three other, very rare types of cancer are not to be covered here.

Diseases of the gallbladder

Since the gallbladder is a reserve facility for special stress, its failure due to disease or surgical removal is an added stress on the liver. Therefore, it must be included in any therapy of the liver.

Roughly every fifth person in the USA and in Europe has gallstones (Harrison).

Gallstones
These are crystalline lumps of normal and atypical bile components in wrongly composed bile. Four-fifths contain cholesterol, $\frac{1}{5}$ pigments as the main component. Usually, the cause is poor nutrition (cf. the chapter on scientific basics). They do not occur in vegans, and are much rarer in vegetarians. Certain medications may promote the formation of gallstones. They can be shown in ultrasound in 95 % of cases.

Gallstones, which are invisible to x-rays, can be slowly dissolved by medication using the cholesterol-dissolving cheno-desoxycholic acid and similar substances, with diarrhoea and other side effects. Without further measures, however, 30–55 % of cases will see a recurrence of gallstones after 3–12 years.

More often, the gallstones are broken up by extracorporeal pressure surges. This is only possible with stones that appear in x-ray images, where the gallbladder is otherwise healthy and where there are no more than 3 stones. Under these conditions, the treatment will work in 95 % of cases. Side effects occur from the discharge of stone fragments: gallbladder colic in $\frac{1}{3}$ of cases and pancreatitis or gallbladder inflammation in about every hundredth patient.

Gallbladder inflammation
Acute gallbladder inflammation is usually a consequence of occlusion of the exit of the gallbladder by a stone. Much less often, it occurs from infection rising from a chronically clogged, diseased intestine. This condition must be carefully determined by diagnosis.

The feared *gallbladder colic* occurs when a stone is caught in the discharge duct of the gallbladder or the bile duct, with increased pressure in the gallbladder, which uselessly contracts under massive pain. The pain usually occurs in waves that are perceived below the right costal arch and often radiate into the right shoulder. Between the colic, the feeling of pressure in the upper abdomen continues, typically radiating up between the shoulder blades. Often, there will be vomiting.

Gallbladder colic is a medical emergency and is usually treated with relaxing and pain-relieving medication.

Our therapy of first choice is neural therapy that reflexively stimulates the skin areas connected to the gallbladder, not only relieving the colic but also thoroughly calming the resulting gallbladder inflammation. Acupuncture and homeopathy or skilful connective-tissue massage of the painful zone can also be used sensibly. After this, further medical follow-up is required.

During the colic, complete fasting and no more than some sips of warm peppermint or chamomile tea are permitted. Then therapy for the gallbladder inflammation starts.

Chronic gallbladder inflammation may continue all the way to suppuration (gallbladder empyema). This condition usually develops slowly, flaring up acutely when there is a special stress or exhaustion. More often than acute gallbladder inflammation, it develops from rising infection from a chronically ill, clogged intestine. The inflammation may very easily continue from the gallbladder into the bile ducts of the liver. Therefore, quick and intense care is mandatory right after discovery of a gallbladder inflammation; it is just as important to care for the intestine prophylactically, study its bacteria milieu and adjust it.

General therapeutic notes
For all liver and gall diseases, treatment of the intestine is a central therapeutic measure. Both constipation and diarrhoea are signs of chronic gastro-intestinal diseases. Usually, years of constipation have already passed. Then follows the next degree of inflammation of the large intestine, chronic diarrhoea. Here, the entire intestine has lost its fine selection and resorption capacity and empties its contents explosively and loaded with inflammation elements and toxins. All sections of the gastrointestinal channel are coordinated with each other subtly in their function in the form of reaction chains of micro-molecular hormones. The acid and enzyme production of the stomach and the production of the digestive juices and enzymes of the pancreas and duodenum will slowly decline and result in constipation.

The healthy intestine should easily discharge soft but shaped stools at least once, but usually two or three times per day, without cramps or lots of gases or mucous. Hard, dark stool suggests incipient intestinal putrefaction and inertia.

The change of the order of meals, with fruit at the beginning and lots of raw food and vegetables, will usually be enough to overcome this inertia without further measures. With a diet of such rich raw vegetable food, the stool will have an ochre to light-yellow colour, which should not be mistaken for the clay-grey colour of the jaundice stool. The food parts are digested. The light yellow suggests active, effective, unused bile.

Further suggestions for intestinal regulation can be found in the chapter "The healing plan". They must be observed and carried out in the treatment outlined here.

For gallbladder inflammation, bile excretion must be examined by probing at the connection point of the bile duct to the duodenum and the pathogens must be isolated and disinfected. Amoebae, which have retreated to the gallbladder after an intestinal infection and thus have escaped anti-parasite therapy, will often be found as the cause. The bile is removed with the duodenal probe to clean the bile ducts. Whether there are gallstones or other causes must be determined precisely. Only precise knowledge of the individual situation permits development of treatment. Therefore, we can only suggest general directives here, rather than provide details for care. Information on nutrition can be found in the chapter "The healing plan" and in the diet stages II and III.

Excitement and sudden effort should be avoided. They may cause relapses. Strong cooling or overheating is to be avoided as well. Good, medium warming of the liver should be observed.

Lots of movement every day (long walking, later hiking) is important to stimulate the activity of the gallbladder, bile ducts, intestine and breathing. Daily connective-tissue massage of the reflex zones, the skin areas that belong to the gallbladder, may be very useful in relaxing and better emptying the gallbladder. Oil treatment is described on page 72. Neural therapy and skilful phytotherapy are effective for complete healing. Classic homeopathy or acupuncture can be valuable as well.

A feared but fortunately rare complication of gallbladder inflammation and stones is partial death of the gallbladder with peritonitis.

Gallbladder carcinoma

Gallbladder carcinoma is four times more common in women than in men. Ninety percent of these patients have gallstones. Chronic gallbladder inflammation is considered an important partial cause. Another cause is the "porcelain gallbladder", which is caused by lime precipitation in the gallbladder. It must be removed.

Bile-duct stones (choledocholithiasis)

About 15 % of patients with gallstones, and among older patients even 25 %, experience discharge of larger gallstones into the main bile duct (ductus choledochus). Two complications are feared:

The inflammation of the large bile duct (cholangitis)
This is a rising infection from the intestine when there are stones in the large bile duct. It may occur acutely, with sudden high fever peaks, chills and gallbladder-colic pain. This bacterial infection is dangerous, since it may cause a potentially fatal general infection of the blood with abscess formation in the liver and elsewhere (sepsis). In addition to immediate antibiotic therapy, surgical treatment is required.

Cholangitis may also occur chronically.

Jaundice from occlusion of the bile duct (occlusion icterus) If jaundice occurs slowly without strong symptoms, a carcinoma must be excluded as the cause at once.

If it occurs suddenly, with gallbladder colic, it is usually an occlusion from a stone. Eyes and skin become very yellow, the urine turns dark and the stool pale and light. Again, immediate medical aid, diagnosis and therapy are required.

In cases of gallbladder and bile-duct stones and inflammation, there is often also pancreatitis.

Postcholecystectomy syndrome

Nearly one-third of patients whose gallbladder has been surgically removed continue to suffer from unpleasant gallbladder pain that is not dissimilar to their symptoms before surgery. This pain is caused by interferences in the inner and outer surgical scars and may continue for years or even decades. The affected patients are often misunderstood. The pain is considered psychosomatic and the patient is sent to psychotherapy, which of course cannot be effective at all.

The treatment of choice is neural therapy. These patients are often permanently symptom free after the first interference treatment.

Plant remedies for liver-gall diseases (phytotherapy, spagyrics)

There are many liver remedies that are offered as entirely harmless. We urge you to discuss medication with your doctor carefully. The diversity of liver functions requires careful selection that must be closely coordinated with you.

For a number of herbs that we used to call "amara" (bitters), contents and effectiveness have been clearly documented in the last few years. These includes *milk thistle (Silybum marianum)*, which has a **liver-cell-protecting effect** and therefore should already be given during the acute phase of hepatitis. Milk thistle has no side effects and is extraordinarily well tolerated. Preparation as a tea: Rx *Fructus Cardui Mariae*: pour hot water over 1 teaspoon, let it seep for 15 minutes and drink hot in small sips, 1 cup each on an empty stomach in the morning, 30 minutes before lunch and before going to bed at night.

The effect of the *artichoke* is a little less **cell-protecting but more bile-stimulating**. It can always be taken as artichoke syrup (Holle).

Wormwood (Artemisia absinthum) has a **carminative (anti-flatulent) gallbladder-stimulating** effect and also stimulates the mind. Larger amounts of wormwood, however, have a very stimulating effect on the central nervous system and are therefore poisonous. Therefore absinthe is forbidden in many countries. Wormwood tea, however, contains the suitable amount of effective substances and can be used in reasonable amounts. Wormwood is also valuable for its **peristaltic-promoting effect in the upper abdomen** (stomach, bile ducts).

Goldenseal (Curcuma longa or domestica) comes from Java and has a **strong gallbladder-stimulating effect:** Rx *Rhiz. curcumae* conc. 200.0. Briefly boil 1 tablespoon in 1 glass of water 3× per day and drink it in small sips. It can be mixed with peppermint.

Celandine (Chelidonium majus)

Relieves cramps in the bile ducts. *Fumitory (Fumaria officinalis)* mostly has a **gallbladder-stimulating** effect and is available as a lozenge. Its effect can be valuable in the jaundice stage.

Radish (Raphanus sativus) does not have a gall-stimulating effect but **drives intestinal peristalsis** and thus is an important and old remedy for liver diseases. It can either be enjoyed in fine slices throughout the day or drunk as fresh juice (1 dl/day) over many days.

Dandelion (Taraxacum officinale) contains a large number of effective substances that **stimulate liver metabolism**. The taproot and herb must be used. It is harmless and can be applied for an extended period of time: Rx *Radix taraxaci cum herba* S: 1–2 teaspoons per one cup of water, boil briefly and steep for 15 minutes.

Lavender (Lavendula officinalis) has a stimulating effect on **bile formation and bile flow**. At the same time, it calms the mind, which effect can also be achieved by dripping the pure essential oil onto the pillow. Lavender blossoms are plants and effective as a tea.

Spagyric essences and tinctures contain alcohol and therefore should be avoided in the highly acute stage of hepatitis or liver poisoning.

Traditional Chinese medicine generally knows the same remedies and effects. It differs in the type of considerations that lead to prescription and that refer to observations of the patient's condition. For the knowledgeable doctor, they are an important aid in choosing the right herbal recipe. However, we currently have to warn against complete, complex and supposedly Chinese finished products, which must be clearly differentiated from reliable traditional Chinese phytotherapy.

Much the same can be said about Tibetan phytotherapy.

Treatment of infections

Since the common pharmaceutical flu treatments usually stress the liver and only act on the symptoms, they must be avoided in liver diseases. The challenge of an infection is an opportunity to regenerate and strengthen the immune system for the body if it is strong enough to react with fever, intense circulation of the entire organism, thirst, sweat and strong activation of the entire metabolism and immune- cell formation that serves to eliminate the pathogens.

For example, the interferon discussed in hepatitis therapy is only one of many substances formed by the infected body's white blood cells; under high fever, the body doses it masterfully and uses it without side effects.

Symptomatic fever reduction by anti-inflammatory medication in infections acts by its inhibition of formation of prostaglandins, other substances of the body that increase the immune response, in a kind of sabotage of the healing efforts of the organism. Such treatment should usually be avoided. The lack of effectiveness of fever-reducing "flu remedies" such as salicylic acid, Paracetamol, etc. in terms of healing also has been scientifically proven.

If there is no heart disease and the function of the liver permits heat application (pleasant feeling), an immediate and subsequent overheating bath is very effective. In cases of hepatitis or critical liver function, this treatment should be discussed with your doctor beforehand. The organism's reaction capacity can be improved by a fruit- and vegetable-juice treatment during the acute stage and by suitably chosen spagyric essences.

For therapy of infectious diseases, the following procedure has often proven effective:

1) Immediate preparation of an infusion of linden blossoms (sweat-promoting) in the thermos jug, mixed with fresh lemon juice and flower honey. Drink 3 litres per day.
2) After having drunk at least ½ litre, prepare the first overheating bath at once if possible: run a full bath at 38°C, mix in 5 drops of thyme essence well, measure the temperature, get into the bath and slowly increase to 41°C, remaining in the bath at this temperature for 10 minutes if possible (measure several times). Then lie in a bed previously well lined with bath towels without standing any longer than necessary (danger of dizziness) and without drying off, wrap yourself in the towels and cover yourself well. Under heat and intense circulation of the entire body and massive sweating for approx. ¾ hours, the body will

deal with the infection immediately in many cases. Otherwise, if the treatment is well tolerated, repeat the bath every day until you are well. After sweating, briefly wash with a cold wash cloth and rest (in case of heart diseases, inflammatory liver-gallbladder diseases and progressed liver cirrhosis, always discuss treatment with your attending physician first.)

Spagyric essences and essential oils for treating infections
Add 25 drops of a spagyric tincture of *Echinacea purpurea* or, even better, *angustifolia* in approx. 1 dl lukewarm water. Add 2 drops of tea-tree oil (*Melaleuka altemifolia*), followed by 5 drops of pure medicinal thyme essence and 3 drops of pure peppermint essence (*Menta piperita*). The essences will float on top because they cannot mix with water.

For a weak cold, this mix is used for gargling three times a day in small sips and then swallowed. For a severe cold, repeat 5× per day.

Children under 6 years of age must not take these plant essences. Children over 6 years and up to 35 kg receive half the dose, older children the full one.

Echinacea (coneflower) strengthens the immune response. The oily essences increase this effect, treat the mucous membranes and also directly fight viruses and bacteria.

Echinacea (Madaus), Echinaforce (Bioforce), Spagymun (Spagyros) and others can be used as well. A similar, ready-mixed preparation of essential oils with outstanding effect is Spagyrom (Spagyros).

Spagyric essences contain alcohol. In spite of the very low amount, it is better for patients with liver damage or hepatitis to drip the essence mix on a small piece of sugar, let the alcohol evaporate and then suck the sugar bit by bit and swallow it.

Hydrotherapy

In the inflammatory stage, cold applications are usually indicated. Often, one can feel whether cold or heat is better (Winternitz, 1877).

Long-term cold compresses are anti-inflammatory only in the highly acute stages. A brief gush of cold water stimulates circulation and leads to deep inner heating, provided that the body part to be gushed and the entire body are previously well warmed. Only after a thorough heating in the shower, bath or with dry brushing of the skin can cold pours have a beneficial effect. If you feel weak, be careful and do not apply too much cold stimulus.

In the acute stage of local inflammations, washes with a cold rag, cool compresses with white cabbage leaves or quark or cold gushes of 1 second have a positive effect after sufficient previous warming.

If the inflammation is already much less acute (less hot), partial or full baths with 10 drops of pure lavender or juniper essence can be very pleasant since they stimulate circulation of the diseased tissue. The bath may be completed with a brief cold gush of water to stimulate circulation.

In case of non-inflammatory, rheumatic or gallbladder pain, a hot compress (steam compress) or the application of a hay flower bag has a positive effect. For all compresses, it is necessary to place a moisture-tight plastic or rubber layer around the wrapped body part and a wool blanket above. Wet and cold compresses should be left on until the treated body region starts a strong inner heating. Warm compresses should be removed before they cool. The treated region is then wrapped warmly and the entire body is covered warmly.

After all water applications, rest for ½ to ¾ hour lying down. All effects of one treatment should have ended before the next one is started.

Compresses

(Thüler, 1986; Spengler, 1969; Eichler, 1981)

Body compress
(according to Kuhne and Priessnitz)

Indication: stimulation of the entire digestive system and the liver in liver diseases, metabolism problems, digestive problems, flatulence, constipation, sleeping problems, menopausal complaints, nervousness.

First place on the bed a woollen blanket that should reach from the neck to the feet. Place a 1 m wide rubber or plastic cloth above it crosswise.

Now fold a linen cloth to 1×2 metres and place it across the woollen blanket. This is the envelope for the poultice. It should reach from the armpits to the knees. If the blankets are not pre-heated (tumbler dryer), the patient lies on them and folds them around himself until they become warm. Now open the blankets again. The patient sits up or gets out of bed briefly.

37

The actual compress cloth should be approx. 160×180 cm (linen is better than cotton). It is folded to 80 cm and put in cold water, wrung out briefly and quickly spread across the cotton blanket in the middle. The patient lies on it at once so that the cloth reaches from his armpits to the groin. The legs are placed together and the arms are held up. He should now inhale and briefly hold his breath (this makes the cold stimulus feel pleasant!). Fold in the compress cloth and then the dry cotton cloth closely and without wrinkles around the patient at once. Place his arms along his sides. Now the patient is closely wrapped in the woollen blanket from the armpits to the feet and covered in a warm blanket. The entire procedure must be performed quickly.

Let the patient rest for 1½–3 hours like this with the window opened. If he falls asleep, the can also leave the compress on much longer, but no longer than until it has become hot and dry.

The loin compress
This is performed precisely like the body compress but only from the upper abdomen to the thigh. The stimulus is less strong on the liver and more on the abdominal organs.

The neck compress
This compress works well for inflammatory diseases of the throat or glands. In the same procedure, it is placed around the neck approx. 20 cm wide.

The leg compress
This compress helps against sleeping problems. It is placed around the calves at a width of 60 cm, better separately around each lower leg. The stimulus is even less than from the loin compress.

Gushes

This is usually done with cold water that should run freely from an approx. 1.5 m long hose. The ideal hose thickness is ¾ inch, but a shower-head hose can be used as well.

The full gush
Indication: Stimulates regulation of the circulation, metabolism and bile formation.

Remove the shower head from the bathtub or shower (use the free hose end). A full gush is strongly stimulating.

The well-heated patient stands in the tub or shower with his back to the water jet. The helper pours a weak, wide water jet on him: starting at the back of the right foot, quickly up the outside of the leg to the buttocks and back down to the heel on the inside. Then the left leg is gushed the same way. Now move up from the right little finger to the shoulder and neck. Stay there for 5 seconds so that one-third of the jet runs down the front and two-thirds down the back. Then repeat the same on the left arm. Now the patient turns with the back to the wall and the same gush is repeated on the front of the legs, arms and shoulders.

Leg gush
Indication: Regulation problems of the circulation (orthostatic circulation weakness), varicose diseases, arterial circulation problems of the legs, problems falling asleep, digestion problems.

Proceed as for the full gush, but treat only the legs. End the gush with the sole of the foot on both sides.

The alternating leg gush
Indication: problems falling asleep (it reduces blood pressure and reduces anxiety).

First perform the leg gush as above on both sides with the jet at approx. 38°. Stay in the groin for about 8 seconds until it is well warmed. Then perform the leg gush on both sides cold.

The alternating knee gush
Indication: cold feet, inflammation of the bile ducts, jaundice, constipation, sleeplessness.

Proceed as for the alternating leg gush, but stay at the small toe at the front, stay above the knee cap for 8 seconds (until warmed) and go back down on the inner side, then perform the same on the other leg and end on both sides from the front by staying above the knee cap.

Then repeat the same gush quickly from the front and rear with cold water. Again stay for 5–8 seconds. This leads to pleasant inner warming.

The abdominal gush
(according to Winternitz)
Indication: digestion problems, abdominal problems, prostate conditions.

This treatment increases and expands the stimulation of the leg gush. It is performed the same way, but the insides of the thighs are treated for longer and the jet stays on the abdomen for approx. 8 seconds. The general previous heating is particularly important here. Again, lie down afterwards and wrap yourself warmly. This will stimulate the pelvic organs wonderfully.

Kuhne's rubbing hip bath
Indication: diseases and weakness of the pelvic organs (bladder, sexual organs, women's complaints, prostate complaints, rectal complaints).

First, sit in a hot half bath, with the lower legs on a stool placed in the bath tub so that only your pelvis is in the water.

Then empty the bath tub, sit on the stool, place a bucket of cold water in front of you and apply cold water to the inside of your thighs and perineum repeatedly by slapping with a cold bath towel submersed in it. Start above the knees and treat your thighs moving upwards and finally the perineum. There should be a strong reddening of the skin and pleasant inner warming. Then lie in bed warmly wrapped.

Water treading
Indication: problems falling asleep, but also after waking up at night, anxiety, fatigue on hikes, varicose veins, mild arterial circulation problems, problems with heat regulation, tendency to hypertension, functional heart problems, bad headache.

Place a tub filled with cold water to approx. 40 cm next to your bed. If you cannot sleep, sit on the edge of your bed and put your feet in the tub, then step in this bath for ½–1 minute standing or sitting, dry your feet and lie down. Water treading in a mountain brook is particularly pleasant. Even dew treading in a cold, moist meadow in the early morning is similar in its effect.

The baths

The overheating bath
Indication: fever, to strengthen the fever reaction of the body, to strengthen the immune response to infections, hepatitis, bile-duct inflammation, cancer. Counterindication: discuss with your doctor beforehand if you have a heart condition.

First, drink 2–3 litres of linden-blossom tea with fresh lemon juice and a little honey from a thermos jug. Then place wide bath towels across your bed.

Fill the bath tub with lukewarm water and add 3 drops of pure thyme essence. Then lie in the tub and let hot water run in until it reaches 41° C. Keep this temperature by letting more water run in for 10 minutes. Then immediately (caution: danger of dizziness when standing up) lie in the prepared bed and wrap yourself in bath towels. Covered in warm blankets, sweat covered for 30–45 minutes. Then briefly wash cold and rest.

The cold half-bath
(according to Winternitz, Kuhne, Kneipp)

Indication: gallstones, sleeping problems, digestion problems, flatulence, constipation.

After thorough warming, slowly enter the bath tub and sit in the cold water, which should reach your navel. Inhale deeply! Stay in the cold water for 6–10 seconds (later increase gradually to 1 minute), dry off well at once and lie down to rest warmly covered. According to Dr Winternitz, this bath, supplemented by a moving cold gush of the abdomen, improves portal-vein circulation.

The three-quarters bath
Indication: calming, tension, sleeping problems.

Bath additive: 10 drops of pure lavender essence or balm essence. Bath temperature: approx. 38° C. The water level should be to the nipple. Stay for approx. 10 minutes. Then take a brief cool shower and rest covered up well for at least 20 minutes.

Alternating arm bath
Indication: headache, circulation problems.

Fill sink with well-heated water and strongly heat your arms in it to the middle of the upper arms; you should be well warmed at the beginning.

Now drain the water and fill the sink with very cold water. Submerse both arms for 10–15 seconds until you feel a painful cold. Then swing the arms until you feel a strong inner warming. Rest.

Alternating foot bath
Indication: bile duct inflammation, jaundice, cold feet, sleeping problems, flatulence.

Place 2 large buckets next to each other, fill one with very warm, the other with very cold water and sit in front of them.

First submerse your feet and lower legs in the warm water for 5 minutes, then in the cold one for 10–15 seconds. Put feet into warm stockings at once and rest warmly covered.

Alternating shower
Indication: sleeping problems, regulation weakness of the circulation (difficulty getting up, lack of appetite in the morning).

First shower very warm for 5 minutes, then very briefly cold, then rub dry. Dress warmly at once.

Washes

Body wash
Indication: digestion problems (intestinal inertia, flatulence), problems falling asleep. Caution: for bladder infections, use the overheating bath.

You should be well warmed first. Prepare a tub with cold water and a terrycloth rag. Start with the moist rag in the area of the appendix and revolve it to below the breast in a clockwise motion 20–40 times. Re-moisten the rag several times. Then rest warmly covered.

The full wash
Indication: improves defences, regulation weakness of the circulation and the heat balance, promotes skin circulation and stimulates the inner organs, for chronic rheumatic diseases, nervousness and sleeping problems.

For bile duct inflammation or jaundice, we recommend adding vinegar (expansion of the skin vessels) with 1 part vinegar to 2 parts water (according to Dr Spengler).

Procedure: outside and inside the right arm to the armpit, repeat on the left, then throat, chest, body, back, right leg outside and inside, then rear, from the buttocks down, repeat on the left; finally both foot soles in sequence.

This wash should be done quickly, and the rag should be put back into the cool water repeatedly; do not dry off at once (evaporation coldness). Then dry off briskly and rest warmly covered.

Abdominal wash
Indication: intestinal inertia, flatulence. Caution: for urinary-tract infection use the overheating bath.

Proceed as for the whole wash but wash only the abdomen.

Compresses and applications

The steam compress according to Kneipp
Indication: this treatment relaxes the muscles. Colic and cramps of inner organs, flatulence, liver-gallbladder pain, digestion problems or muscle tension.

Procedure: a folded linen cloth of suitable size is submersed in boiling water (caution: danger of burns). The cloth is taken from the water with a tool, placed in terrycloth, wrung in it and folded in a flannel cloth for a compress, which is placed on the area to be treated when it is no longer perceived as too hot on the upper arm, and wrapped with an elastic bandage. Once the compress has cooled, it is removed. Then continue with at least one hour of bed rest.

The hot liver compress
Indication: the heat has a cramp-relieving effect and stimulates the liver circulation, bile flow and liver metabolism in digestion problems.

Pour ½ litre of boiling water over 1 teaspoon yarrow and let it steep for 3–5 minutes. Now place a wool wrapping cloth that will enclose the body behind the back of the sitting patient. A cotton cloth is folded in 6 layers to 60×70 cm, soaked with the yarrow tea, placed in a dry terrycloth and wrung out well. The drier it is wrung, the better, because the compress can be applied hotter and will stay warm for longer. Slightly slap the compress on the skin above the liver several times and then apply quickly. Place a rubber or plastic foil around it and attach the wool wrap closely over it. The compress should be left for ½–1 hour. Then rest for ½ hour.

The hot roll
Indication: weakness of digestion, flatulence, to stimulate the liver, nervousness, sleep problems.

Fold 2 terrycloths lengthwise and roll them in very closely and slightly offset above each other so that they form a kind of spiral-shaped tip at one end. On the other end, they form a kind for funnel. Roll two more terrycloths around it so that the funnel does no longer grow any deeper. Now pour 1 litre of boiling water into the funnel of the roll. If it has been coiled closely enough, it will take up all water and no water will drip back out. Now wrap this roll with a fifth terrycloth so that it will protrude by approx. 20 cm on both ends, which you can hold with both hands as you would a rolling pin. Now roll it gently with a massaging motion over the liver area and then clockwise over the belly. The skin should become hot and reddened. You can also apply this treatment yourself easily.

The hay flower bag
Indication: gallstones, non-inflammatory cramps of the upper abdomen; stimulation of the circulation of the liver, bile and portal vein flow and liver metabolism.

It is called the "morphine of herbal treatment": The hay flower bag consists of a blossom mixture of grasses and flowers from a healthy meadow or what remains in the hayloft after the hay is taken away. The application of hay flower has been retained in the general rheumatology of university hospitals.

The essential oils of hay flowers have a simulating effect on the skin circulation and thus also stimulate organ systems that are reflexively connected to the skin area to be treated. Hay flower is a good bath additive. However, its effect is most intense when the hay flowers are directly applied in a small bag. The temperature should be adjusted to the patient's wish and it should be applied every day for 1–2 hours. People who are allergic to grass pollen cannot apply the bags themselves, but can usually tolerate them well when moistly applied. Hay flowers can be bought in the pharmacy and placed in a gauze napkin or the bags can be bought ready-made. They are infused with hot water for heating and placed on the liver or belly once the temperature is bearable. Apply a moisture-tight layer above and then a wool cloth.

Belly massage (according to Winternitz)
Indication: constipation from intestinal inertia, flatulence.

The patient lies relaxed on the back or the left side. Start on the right abdomen and continue the massage clockwise along the course of the large intestine to the left abdomen. Reach into the abdominal wall gently but deeply with both hands and move the enclosed tissue gently, shaking and swinging.

Description of some water applications and compresses

Indication table:

Diseases	Application
liver-gallbladder diseases	body compress, full gush, alternating foot bath, full wash, steam compress according to Kneipp
flatulence	body compress, cold half bath, alternating foot bath, body wash, abdominal wash, steam compress according to Kneipp
sleep problems	body compress, leg gush, alternating leg gush, alternating knee gush, three-quarters bath, alternating foot bath, body wash, water treading, cold half bath, alternating shower, full wash
weak circulation, hypotension	leg compress, full gush, leg gush, water treading, alternating shower, full wash
digestion problems	body compress, leg gush, abdominal gush, Kuhne's rubbing hip bath (rectum), cold half bath, body wash, abdominal wash, steam compress according to Kneipp

Diseases	Application
constipation	body compress, alternating knee gush, cold half bath, abdominal wash
varicose disease	leg gush, water treading
arterial circulation problems	leg gush, water treading
cold feet	alternating knee gush, alternating foot bath
inflammation of the bile ducts	alternating knee gush
menopausal problems	body compress
jaundice	alternating knee gush, alternating foot bath, full wash (with added vinegar)
abdominal problems, prostate problems, women's complaints	loin compress, Kuhne's rubbing hip bath
proctitis (inflammation of the rectum)	Kuhne's rubbing hip bath
heat regulation problems	full wash
blood pressure, tending to be too high	water treading
heart problems, functional	full wash
strengthening the body's defences	Kuhne's rubbing hip bath, full wash
gallstones	cold half bath
nervousness	three-quarters bath
headache	water treading, alternating arm bath
lack of appetite in the morning (difficulty getting up)	alternating shower
hard muscle tension	three-quarters bath, steam compress according to Kneipp
colic and cramps of inner organs	full wash, steam compress according to Kneipp
liver-gall pain	full wash, steam compress according to Kneipp
liver diseases	body compress
inflammation of the throat, angina	neck compress
prostate problems	abdominal gush, Kuhne's rubbing hip bath

Homeopathic therapy, miasmatically inherited consequences of diseases and traumas

Homeopathy is based on the discovery of Samuel Hahnemann that certain physical procedures permit the release of immaterial medicinal effects from matter. By means of step-by-step dilution and massive mechanical shaking, specific information for the original substance is saved in the energetic structure of the alcohol molecule or sugar molecule and made durable.

Homeopathic medication is comparable to a kind of programme disc that – similar to computer technology – permits entering ordering information into the human organism. The homeopathic medicinal effect is not material, i.e. it does not directly manipulate the biochemical processes as a molecule or substance, but in a higher way, as an ordering impulse on an electromagnetic path.

This is where the ingenious minds of Bircher-Benner and Samuel Hahnemann meet. Bircher researched the non-material ordering effect of raw fresh vegetable food on chronic diseases in decades of clinical work, while Hahnemann released non-material ordering information from substances and observed their effects on the healthy and finally the sick human.

The homeopathic medicinal effect is highly specific. Only the medication that would produce the symptoms in a healthy person can cause the healing (ordering) impulse for what is to be healed in the patient. Therefore a precise collection of symptoms and basic understanding of the personality and current mood of the patient are an absolute prerequisite for finding the right medication. The wrong medication will do nothing, the almost-right one almost nothing; if the medication is just right, it often starts up enormous self-healing powers in the organism.

Homeopathy is a very valuable aid in treatment of chronic diseases and particularly of liver-gallbladder diseases, even though it will not remove the cause of the disease on its own. Homeopathic therapy without concurrent reorganisation of the nutrition and lifestyle of the patients often permits the experienced classically homoeopathic practitioner to cause visible relief, and in earlier stages also sometimes healing of some liver conditions; however, it does not remove the causes: faulty nutrition, intestinal putrefaction, overload of the connective tissue with metabolic harmful substances, overload of the regulating structures of the organism (basic substance of the soft connective tissue), through which the energetic ordering impulses are conducted (Pischinger, Heine, 1991). Thus the disease continues again even after the condition has improved. The homeopathic doctor knows that the entirety of destructive influences of faulty nutrition, irritants and stimulants, alcohol, harmful substances and a lifestyle that does not observe the day/night rhythm cannot be countered.

On the other hand, experience shows that many, partially severe forms of the liver-gallbladder diseases can be healed by consistent application of the ordering and nutritional therapy set up by Bircher-Benner. For the order therapy of the disease in the clinic, homeopathy is a very valuable help, particularly where the ordering impulse of homeopathic medication is able to bring the severely ill person out of a critical situation and to guide the decompensated regulation processes in a healing direction so that the self-healing powers can start up quickly and the order therapy is able to unfold its full effect at once.

A second indication for classic Homeopathy is miasmatic stress. From the homeopathic point of view, this means constitutional weaknesses that are the inherited consequences of wrongly treated diseases or unhealed physical or mental traumas of ancestors. Such constitutional weaknesses are usually visible from birth, but may also appear much later, e.g. as panic in specific situations or phobias, the cause of which cannot be explained from the personal biography even with precise knowledge of the earliest childhood, e.g. acquired from psychoanalysis. An exact understanding of the feeling during anxiety conditions and during dreams of the patient permits very precise choice of methods. Purely physical miasmatically inherited weaknesses do not actually exist, even though they are consequences of inherited diseases. Thousands of healing processes have shown that *with every disappearance of physical symptoms, mental contents emerge in the consciousness* which had belonged to the previously disturbed life energy. For example, war threats appear in dreams of people who never experienced war and never deal with war stories or war movies, even in young children. Miasmatically inherited traumas may originate centuries ago. We differentiae clearly between them and mental contents of the collective unconscious (C. G. Jung, 1964, 1970, 1971), which probably represent the general experience of mankind that has entered the genetic code over the ages, such as dream images of dragons (dinosaurs). *The collective subconscious* is general and present in the same manner in every person, while the miasmatic burden is strictly individual, applies to only one person and must be healed in precisely this person in order not to be passed on again.

The diversity of the possible homeopathic medications for one and the same diagnosis corresponds to the eternal diversity of human individuality. Treatment is not targeted at the disease, but the individual impairment of the physical, mental and spiritual personality of the patient. Anamnesis and therapy thus become a fascinating exploratory journey for the patient and doctor that, if properly guided by the doctor, will cause a deeper understanding and awareness of the patient of his personality and disease. The insights acquired in this manner at the same time form the ideal basis for planning the entire order therapy, which can in no case be replaced by homeopathic therapy for healing chronic diseases to achieve true, permanent healing.

The new scientific acupuncture

Acupuncture is one of the oldest methods for stimulating and guiding the regulation activity of the organism. In the last few years, it has already received a fairly solid scientific basis in many examples of basic research (König and Wancura, 1989; Heine, 1990 and many more). In its thousands of years of research into therapeutic effects, Chinese medicine has shown how the individual organs, muscle groups and body layers are interconnected. These insights precisely match the neurophysiological knowledge of our western medicine, but exceed it by far. According to Chinese medicine, outer (e.g. climate and seasonable) influences and inner factors such as stress on the mind may cause our basic regulation to lose its manifold balance, and thus cause diseases.

The meridians are – as therapeutic experience has shown – inner connection tracks by which the acupuncture points are connected. We can view them as the main conductors of the connective-tissue-like basic regulation system (Pischinger and Heine, 1990). The anatomic structure of the acupuncture points has been documented impeccably by Heine (1990).

Acupuncture has proven its worth as a constitutional readjustment method in liver-gallbladder diseases. If it is not effective when properly applied, the foci in the sense of an interference field of neural therapy are at fault. They must be restored.

Neural therapy according to Huneke

Neural therapy is an order-therapeutic adjustment procedure with injections of procaine, a local anaesthetic. Procaine was first produced in the 1920s. A small change to the cocaine molecule from the cola nut completely removed the mood-lifting, addiction-causing active ingredient. There is no euphoria and no addiction to procaine.

Before this synthesis, medicine only knew cocaine as a local anaesthetic for surgical wound treatment. Later, lidocaine, which is still often used in surgery, was synthesised. Neural therapy prefers procaine to lidocaine since it expands vessels (unlike any other local anaesthetic), is excreted directly through the kidneys without stressing the liver and is tolerated without adverse effects even in large doses.

The membrane potential (charge differential) at the cell membranes is decisive for their ability to perform their energetic and metabolic function. The cells of sick, reflexively or energetically stressed tissue zones suffer under a sustained depolarisation of their cell membranes. They do not apply the energy that would be necessary to restore the healthy charge ratios, and have a reflexive negative influence on each other and on other body regions that are connected to them. Inside the cells there is continuous faulty metabolism, with collection of unprocessed degradation products. The stressed tissue is over-acidified, hardened, charged electrically as compared to healthy tissue and usually painful. It becomes an energetic interference for other body areas or organs connected to it, which show symptoms of functional impairment or pain as a consequence.

An organism that is stressed by several such interference fields may often tolerate the interference for a long time and compensate for it. If new interference fields are added, it will, however, slowly lose its ability to regulate and become ill as a whole. Often, the phenomenon of the "secondary strike" is observed as well: an accident, acute disease, stressful dental treatment, or often a fateful mental impact causes a general tipping. The acute stress exceeds the organism's ability to compensate; it becomes ill as a whole and falls into a lack of courage and strength, into a deep depression. If one does not know the situation, there is a risk of a wrongly chosen and therefore ineffective treatment, e.g. by psychotherapy or prescription of psychopharmaceuticals. The only continually effective treatment is neural therapy.

By careful, slow and only slightly painful injection of procaine into an interference field, the membranes of all cells of the stressed tissue are completely charged (polarised) for 20 minutes. These 20 minutes of anaesthetic effect of the procaine seal all cells of the interference field completely against any outer influences and stimuli. This relief time is, according to experience, sufficient for their extensive regeneration.

Any sick, non-functional or injured zone of the body is initially an *interference field* that, depending on the body's ability to regulate, will heal completely or only incompletely. Remaining interference fields are foreign bodies and heavy metals (amalgams of the teeth) as well as all chronically ill or incompletely regenerated tissue areas such as scars, dental root granulomas and inflammation foci. A whole sick organ can become an interference field and, in case of an ill liver or gallbladder, cause migraine attacks, so that its accumulated, blocked energy tends to discharge periodically along the meridians and blood vessels towards the head. Other typical interference-field-related diseases include neuralgias that tend to disappear suddenly and permanently if the responsible interference fields are treated.

The treatment of scarring from tonsil surgeries will often cause menstruation problems to disappear, or end childlessness, since the pituitary gland – separated by a tender bone lamella – is only millimetres above it; a stubborn irritation with chronic infection of the bladder neck may suddenly be gone after treatment of a heart-surgery scar in front of the sternum. We have already spoken of the strong interference field of the sick intestine for the liver and the disappearance of the "postcholecystectomy syndrome", the continued gallbladder pain after gallbladder surgery, through the infiltration of the surgery scar with procaine. According to experience, any tiny interference field anywhere in the body may also cause interferences of the parts of the body that are the farthest away from it. If only a single interference field is responsible for a disease, e.g. rheumatic arthritis, the joint pain will disappear immediately upon infiltration with procaine, and this relief will persist for at least one day. This is called a *"secondary phenomenon"*. With re-infiltration of the interference field, the removal of the symptoms will continue for much longer or forever.

Such secondary phenomena are observed several times per year by the neural therapeutic doctor. Usually, there are several important interference fields. In that case, the disease is improved only by treatment of all interference fields, but still continually and permanently.

Neural therapy has become one of the most important regulative and thus order-therapeutic procedures, particularly where the regulation capacity and thus stimulation of the self-healing powers are blocked by multiple interference fields. This is called a *regulation block*. Such people are unable to develop fever in case of infections, will react with extreme sensitivity to weather changes, temperature fluctuations and any outer and inner influences and usually have not only tried all the classic medical therapies and psychotherapies but also a number of regulative therapy attempts without any success until neural therapy finally is able to restart their regulation capacity. Another very valuable method of neutral neural therapy is *segment therapy*. Here, irritation of the skin areas reflexively connected to the inner organs (dermatomes) is used by setting skin welts to regulate the function of the associated organ. We have already mentioned this method for treatment of acute gallbladder colic.

Surgical Procedures

Removal of a gallbladder that cannot be healed (cholecystectomy) has become a minor surgery today because of the endoscopic technique. This procedure also leaves a scarred interference field in the form of the postcholecystectomy syndrome described above, a partial persistence of gallbladder pain that requires neuraltherapeutic aftertreatment. The new surgical technique, however, has decisive advantages and much lower surgery and anaesthesia risks. The removal of such gallbladders is also particularly important since a gallbladder that cannot be healed usually greatly impairs body regulations.

If the liver function is no longer sufficient because of liver cirrhosis, *liver transplants* are used more and more often to save lives today. The liver as a whole is removed and immediately replaced by a donated liver.

This procedure can only be recommended to persons who do not have any other severe chronic diseases. After a transplant, lifelong immunosuppressive therapy (Cyclosporine) is required to prevent the natural rejection reaction of the organism against the foreign donor organ.

Since 1983, the survival chances after a liver transplant have gradually improved. Four-fifths of patients can live another year with the donor organ after surgery, about 60% at least 5 years.

At the moment, about 80% of people who have had a successful liver transplant can return to work at least partially, and there are individual reports of very good progress with truly satisfactory quality of life after the transplant.

The healing plan

Persons suffering from liver and gall diseases are often imbalanced not only physically but also mentally and spiritually. There is a feeling of being insulted, despised. If other people do not treat such people with respect, a particular sensitivity may leave behind feelings of hate, fury or painful bitterness.

This experience, just like even the smallest dietary mistakes, will then often cause a relapse of the liver disease. The former ease is missing, everything becomes difficult, toilsome and too serious. Life becomes a struggle often only fought inside, with possibly offensive persons and with one's own weakness. This grim captivity in a vicious circle about self-respect for one's own person and avoiding relapses, this seemingly hopeless situation, can, however, often be given a beneficial turn by the right healing plan. Experience shows that it is precisely a healing regime that will initiate a decisive way out of this suffering. If performed with care, it will eliminate relapses. The powers of life, ease and joy in life as well as a new, positive attitude will slowly return. This kind of growth can, however, only occur with the patient's return to a natural order of life. The autonomous healing processes embedded in this order increase in intensity.

"A life in the realm of order" was taught by Bircher-Benner. This Hippocratic demand is the greatest help in successful treatment – not a "miracle cure" but a tried and tested, highly effective way to health.

The healing regime

Initially, nutrition is limited to purely vegetarian raw food. This diet is low in fat and free of animal proteins and contains virtually no quickly degradable ("fast") carbohydrates such as are found in bread, other flour-based foods and simple sugar types. This diet gives the liver a very pleasant relief. It can recover in its function every day. This way has turned out to be most reliable for the adjustment.

Completely abstain from irritants such as coffee, black tea, sweets and alcohol, to avoid weakening or even preventing the effect of the raw food. All irritants block the body's regulation and thus prevent the awakening of the self-healing powers. It is easy to stop smoking and alcohol ingestion with skilful medical support. Homeopathy and acupuncture can effectively fight the withdrawal symptoms and support the patient's will – if present. Even the smallest amounts of alcohol have a toxic effect on the liver and must be avoided in any case. The raw-food diet removes waste products, reduces swelling and drains the soft connective tissue; afterwards, in the inter-cellular tissue of the liver and intestine, it can again take up its important mediation and selection task in the nutrition process and detoxification work of the liver, and fulfil its regulatory function.

The increase of the membrane potential of the cells reinforces the living processes of all tissues. The alkaline reserves increase. The central nervous regulation centres recover, as well as the endocrine functions.

The red blood cells recover their elastic properties. The tendency of blood platelets to clot is reduced, "blood-sludge" and vascular diseases are prevented, and oxygen supply to the organs increases, improving their function. The bile recovers its original quality, the environment in the intestine is restored so that the frequent fungal infections disappear and the intestinal mucous membrane grows a healthy micro-flora without which we cannot be healthy. The intestinal mucous membrane is now once again covered by a healthy mucus layer that, with its high content of IG-A antibodies, ensures that the lymph-cell systems of the intestinal mucous membrane can quickly distinguish foreign and body substances, so that no allergy antibodies (IgE) need to be formed.

Thus the frequent allergic reactions of the organism are lessened, and hay fever and eczema improve. The toxins stored in the connective tissue over the years slowly move to the liver and now – after its metabolic function has recovered – can be excreted. This overall regeneration of the organism can be felt clearly even in the first weeks of the diet and increases every day towards new well-being and a feeling of ease. It is truly amazing how an organism starts to blossom under this diet.

Once satisfactory improvement has been achieved after 2–4 weeks of a pure raw-food regime, nutrition can be expanded with the addition of vegetable bouillon, wholemeal mash and cooked, unpeeled potatoes. Often it has proven helpful to alternate this expansion with days of strict raw food, e.g. by enjoying pure raw food on Mondays and Tuesdays and supplementing it with vegetable bouillon and potatoes in the peel from Wednesday to Friday. Only on the weekend will a little wholemeal bread or wholemeal mash be added, supplemented with steamed broccoli, fennel or freshly steamed artichoke. Broccoli and artichokes as well as the spices rosemary and caraway facilitate detoxification of the liver. If good progress continues and if the improvement can be strengthened at a certain level, more additions are permitted: further cooked vegetables, wholemeal bread more often with a little quark with fresh herbs. However, the regime must continue low in salt and fat and rich in fresh food, and remain entirely free of the irritants mentioned above, meat and denatured foods. Relapses mean that the increase was too fast, and the individual diet stages must be performed for longer. Because of the notable improvement in the reactivity of the organism and the overcoming of the healing crises that are possible in the first weeks, patients will experience the surprising healing effect of the diet with relief and joy. The success is inspiring and eases continuation on this path to health.

Below are some suggestions for different forms of treatment for liver-gallbladder diseases, such as hepatitis and gallbladder inflammation.

Treatment of hepatitis

At the first increase in temperature, bed rest and medical treatment are required, since possible complications require immediate action or timely prevention.

Since the bile is pushed back into the blood by inflammation of the liver tissue and the bile ducts and its inflow into the intestine is partially or entirely prevented, the intestine has no bile for digesting fats. Fat therefore must be avoided entirely, at least while the jaundice continues. (Only then and without any heating must small amounts of nut margarine, olive oil, vegetable margarine with a high share of unsaturated oils and only traces of liquid cream be used.)

In the first stage of the disease, all food will be rejected anyway. In this case, warm herbal tea of peppermint or chamomile, sweetened with a very little honey, or unsweetened flatulence or bitter tea is offered. Honey can be administered in small amounts alone, diluted with water. Freshly diluted lemon juice may be added to the tea. It is also often perceived as pleasant when offered pure. Freshly pressed grapefruit or berry juice is also acceptable in spoonfuls. Freshly pressed red or black currant or blueberry juice is particularly beneficial if fresh berries are available. Very finely cut apple slices or germ-free and seedless raisins should also be offered. Raw vegetable juice of carrots, red beet, tomatoes, green leaves, very freshly pressed, right from the juice press, are to be offered as well. Later, add a few lettuce leaves, finely ground carrots and particularly horseradish or radish, witloof and young dandelion.

In addition to the diet, regular emptying of the intestine is important, since intestinal contents without bile tend to putrefy too much. The re-poisoning of the liver from the intestine must be avoided. The stool is a clay grey, which must not be mistaken for the light-yellow healthy stool from a regime rich in raw food! Once the first signs of yellow colouration appear in the stool, the peak of the crisis has been overcome. Then the food should be adjusted to the four regime stages after the acute disease has disappeared. For chronically persisting (continuous) hepatitis B, we particularly recommend using recurring raw-food weeks at intervals.

Intestinal regulation
Apart from chamomile enemas on demand, intestinal emptying must be stimulated by the food and specific additives: lots of raw fresh food, sour dairy products such as butter milk and lean quark, flax seed gruel (see recipe), with added fruit or vegetable juices, or soaked flax seed (2 cups per day), or flax seed flakes of which 3 tablespoons are added to the Bircher muesli. Psyllium seeds (2–3 tablespoons per day) are important as well, one tablespoon 1 hour before meals soaked in warm water. All of these are natural products that stimulate the intestine without causing any mechanical or chemical irritation.

Healing earth (Naturgen, Luvos, Aion A etc.) is also suitable for gentle regulation of intestinal activity. Take 1 heaped teaspoon 1 hour before any meal and, if necessary, again 1–2 teaspoons in the evening. The dosage should be adjusted individually.

Karlsbad salt should only be used according to medical prescription and dosage. It is a great bile duct and intestinal purging agent but can easily act as an irritant and impair the mineral balance if taken in too large quantities or too long.

Karlsbad mineral water (Mühlebrunnen) in contrast has a mild and natural effect and may be taken easily on demand or alternating with the above aids (1 glass in the morning on an empty stomach, lukewarm, in sips). (Also Nürtinger Heinrichsquelle, Staatl. Fachingen and Grenzacher Heilwasser.)

The physical applications, phytotherapy and homeopathic therapy for hepatitis are discussed in the respective chapters.

Treatment of liver cirrhosis

The general rules apply as for hepatitis and diet stages II and III. If the patient is not allergic to milk protein, butter milk, sour milk, kefir, lean quark and natural yoghurt contain valuable proteins (no UHT-products).

Treatment of gallbladder inflammation (cholecystitis)

In addition to the general rules as for hepatitis, take only small amounts of food. Sudden overload of the biliary system must be avoided. Three small main meals with two small interim meals are sufficient, initially according to diet stage II, later a low-fat, stage-III bland diet. Good chewing and salivation are important. Additionally, the suggested herbal teas and gallbladder-stimulating mineral waters, carefully selected, should be drunk copiously. Ice-cooled drinks and alcohol must be avoided. Intestinal activity must be regulated quickly.

To prevent and avoid relapses

No matter how diverse the causes that interact in the occurrence of liver-gallbladder disease, they are in the end all due to impairment of the orders of life. Like the Hippocratic school and Paracelsus before him, Bircher-Benner consistently taught "prevention of the incurable by living in the realm of order."

Most people's lives do not move in the "realm of orders" at all today! Quite the opposite: stress at work, continuous excess of stimulation and impressions, radiation, entertainment, unbalanced foods and drink, irritants, alcohol and medication weaken resistance to diseases over time. A lack of movement, fresh air and sleep also reduce the vital forces. Modern man will hardly find the time for restful hours and creative activity.

There is no miraculous way out of this vicious circle, but only a return to the natural order of life. This truth is simple and open to everyone. Everyone has to accept it on his or her own, however. This insight is particularly important for patients who have overcome a severe liver disease and want to avoid a relapse. Those who want to prevent liver-gallbladder diseases and any chronic illnesses also must understand these connections.

The realm of order starts with the *daily rhythm*. Rise early and go to bed early. If you are not the rare "congenital" night type, you will find with surprise that you feel a lot fresher and better able to perform effectively like this.

The vegetative nervous system is aligned with a circadian rhythm (day and night) in its change between effort and relaxation and is exhausted quickly when night is turned into day and day into night. The natural rhythm also includes a sufficient lunch break with a relaxed lunch and subsequent rest. In the modern working world, however, this lunch break often is no longer possible. Reality gives us an hour's lunch break, with food from the canteen kitchen or a snack stall.

We can free ourselves from these material forces by at least not purchasing junk food or fast food and instead bringing a small, healthful lunch from home (fruits, nuts, bread with raw vegetables and maybe lean quark with fresh herbs or some low-fat cream cheese) that we can eat at the workplace (in summer outdoors). Afterwards, instead of sleeping, we can move around for a quarter of an hour. It is a compromise, but an acceptable solution in a situation that cannot be changed. The main meal in the evening should be taken as early as possible and not contain anything that is difficult to digest.

Body movement is another important subject! Today's people sit too much, move too little. And yet there is a definite trend towards more physical activity in all forms of modern movement such as jogging, mountain biking, snowboarding, skating and so on.

You can also move the "old-fashioned" way and swim, hike, walk or play ball. High-energy sports may suit the modern lifestyle and way of thinking better. However, a regular daily "small" movement programme is more important than a great weekend effort that would stress a non-athlete rather than relax him.

Also regularly practice *conscious breathing*. Deep breathing is very important for circulation of the liver and the kidneys. Lie on your bed, the floor or a reclined chair with the window open, and observe your spontaneous breathing. Then help your respiration by breathing along the spinal cord to the top of your head, and then exhaling down into the abdomen all the way to the toes. On a walk, you can also breathe more consciously. We highly recommend a daily *air bath* of 5 minutes: stand by the open window naked or lie on your balcony or in a hidden shady location in your garden in summer, and massage the skin on your entire body with a dry brush. Sun baths are unfortunately not possible without precautions anymore today. Because the skin will become supple and velvety soft from *sensible sun bathing*, and the entire organism will liven up, you should not dispense with it entirely, but observe the known cautionary measures: light movement is better than motionless "roasting", sun from 11 a.m. to at least 3 p.m. should be avoided, never leave your head uncovered, go for 30 minutes without sunscreen so as to not filter out the vital UVA light, then use crystalline sun blocker. The UVB light is very important for formation of Vitamin D3 and the immune system. In the lower regions below 1000 m. above sea level, it will only come through the atmosphere of the earth in the summer months, but Vitamin D is stored in the liver for winter. Use sun blockers with a high-enough light protection factor. Thirty minutes is entirely sufficient for the healing effect of a sun bath. Take a refreshing shower afterwards.

Water treatments are recommended to liver-gallbladder patients as well. By means of the cold stimulus intensively invigorate the weakened ability to react. The refectory deep inhalation at the first contact with cold water is a valuable breathing stimulus. *Alternating cold and warm showers* are usually well tolerated; they strengthen the body and make you feel comfortable. Increase daily from 1 to 2 and 3 minutes hot and then 20–40 seconds cold, alternating 2–3 times. This treatment will lead to intense reddening of the skin and the disappearance of fatigue. Cold gushes with a strong jet over arms and legs are wonderfully refreshing but only when applied when you are well warmed and have moved enough, never right after getting out of bed.

Alternating warm and cold foot baths help against headache and excessive blood flow into the head. Use two deep buckets, one with water at 39° (to calf height), the other with cold tap water. Put your feet in the hot water for 5–10 minutes, then into the cold water for 10–20–40 seconds, repeat about 3 times. Top up the hot water every time and end with cold water. Sleeping problems can be countered with water treading in a bucket with cold water (12 cm high) or the bath tub. Do not use too-long and too-hot baths.

The *overheating bath* is important to improve circulation and immune defence. This treatment has been described in the chapter on hydrotherapy. The resulting fever and intense arterial circulation are very valuable for the regeneration of the liver. Thorough sweating afterwards leads to additional detoxification through the skin.

Nutrition. For prevention and protection against relapse, persons with liver-gallbladder diseases must return above all to the "realm of the order of life" in terms of nutrition. They need fresh food with fruit, raw vegetables, salads and nuts. At least 50 % and preferably 60–70 % of their food should be raw vegetables, which can be supplemented with wholemeal dishes, vegetables and potatoes and a little fresh milk products. For the dressings on raw vegetables, use only cold-pressed oils with polyunsaturated fatty acids (rapeseed oil, sunflower oil, olive oil, thistle oil, flax seed oil), which have a cholesterol-reducing effect and are antioxidants (cancer protection). A main meal and two simple secondary meals should be enough and the food should be rather on the scant side. Irritants, sweets, white flour dishes, food too rich in fat and protein (meat, cheese!) are to be enjoyed as rare exceptions, not as a daily habit. The craving for such food disappears surprisingly quickly once you have gotten used to the new taste values, especially once you have been rewarded with a new, long-unknown, pleasantly fresh feeling of life. You will no longer feel as if you are actually giving anything up!

Weight should be checked regularly and general condition should be observed. As soon as the weight deviates considerably from the standard upwards or downwards, add a short period of the strict healing regime.

In addition to all of these necessary and helpful measures, you will require a *mental-spiritual alignment*: remembering the essential aspects of life, letting go of the unimportant and over-estimated material values, creative self-realisation, the richness of relationships with the inner and outer world.

Liver patients often feel that they are not respected. Long-past illnesses have often left behind hate and bitterness. Finding new trust in others can be difficult. The disease can only be healed when such trust has been found, however. It is the noble task of medical care for liver patients to help them recover self-respect and trust in others. Constitutional homeopathic therapy can be a great help here. Every active, busy person will also benefit from times of rest, especially when his life is stressful, tense and continually excited and his soul and emotions are neglected.

Today, there are many training options for further mental-spiritual development: autogenic training, yoga, breath training (e.g. "Experienced breathing" according to Middendorf or Zilgrei), Tai Chi, meditative dance, Feldenkrais, therapeutic painting and many others. It may be helpful if a doctor recommends a method to a patient whose physical condition and temperament he knows well, matching his preferences and thus increasing chances of success.

The four diet stages

Diet Stage I
The raw-juice regime

This strict but very effective form of diet can be performed even when fully working but should generally not take more than 1 or 2 days. Later, on the third day, the healing crisis occurs. This is the first changing reaction of the metabolism and the hormonal glands. The reactions are not very pleasant but mark the first awakening of the self-healing forces. Chronic inflammation foci that have often been suppressed for years must again become sensitive to certain degree in order to enable the body to heal the inflammation process.

In liver-gallbladder patients, inflammation foci may appear on the third day of the raw-juice diet. In particular, the often-large interference field of the intestine becomes noticeable. The extended, uninterrupted raw-juice diet is usually reserved for inpatient treatment because of the strong adjustment reaction.

Nevertheless, many severe liver diseases can be successfully treated at home under medical care. For this purpose, the raw-juice diet is performed on Monday and Tuesday, followed by the stage-II diet from Wednesday onwards. This cycle is repeated every week. Even when the patient is working normally, this procedure has proven very helpful. The weekly rhythm of the diet helps set the biologically specified weekly rhythm of healing into motion.

However, if you want to follow a raw-juice diet of several days or weeks at home, you should maintain bed rest and move your body twice per day. This treatment must be supported by a doctor experienced in this method.

The healing crisis:
The frequent sudden drop of insulin demand often causes hypoglycaemic reactions on the third day, such as weakness, dizziness, trembling, palpitations and possibly sweating and fear. They are entirely harmless in everyone who does not have diabetes. Eating raisins that are kept on hand can take care of these symptoms quickly. Headache shows that acidic metabolic products are being flushed from the tissue into the blood stream. Generally, this symptom can be kept within bearable limits by alternating warm and cold arm or foot baths (possibly compresses) until it disappears on its own. Do not take painkillers for the headache!

In the healing crisis of the third raw-juice diet day, there usually also is an emotional impairment that disappears on its own on the fourth day. After a feeling of special well-being around the seventh day, emotional distress almost always returns around the tenth day.

This second distress also is an expression of the starting of a circa-septane (weekly) healing rhythm. Longer than weekly periods mean that the organism cannot find the way to healing because of deeply rooted chronic-disease foci. This situation requires further examination by a doctor trained in this method.

The mood drop of the third juice-regime day usually appears in the form of sadness and anxiety. Think of the advice of C. G. Jung: "Depression is a black lady. Take her to the table and listen to what she has to say!" This is the important moment of mental opening, where the protective wall that we have built up around ourselves for many years to avoid injury, our own surrounding walls and enclosures, start to fall. In this regime phase, there are intense dreams as an expression of incipient healing. All deep dreams, including anxious ones, reflect the healing procedure. There is no need to fear them. With dreams, the soul opens to our consciousness. In our medical practice, we have found that healing of the body is always accompanied by dreams. Do not try to analyse your dreams with symbols. Symbols are not you. They are not individual. Stay still for a moment after waking from a dream instead and ask yourself how you are feeling right then. Not the dream's contents, but the feeling it leaves behind is its true individual meaning. New dreams will bring further answers if you feel your emotions. The raw juice regime has been proven to have a strong anti-depressive effect, which follows the healing crises. Do not be afraid.

Rarely, there may be severe anxiety. In this case, seek appropriate help (person-centred conversational therapy, possibly homeopathic therapy).

Delays of the menstrual cycle under the strict raw-juice regime sometimes occur and may render contraceptives unreliable. Ensure additional safety if contraception is necessary.

Persons living alone should perform their first long-term raw-juice regimes in a clinic. Empathy and understanding of the supporting persons are extremely important for this regime.

The recipes for the raw juice regime are included in the recipe section. Three juice meals with 4–6 dl fresh juice have proven beneficial. The order in which the individual juices are drunk may be chosen instinctively. Enjoy your juices slowly, sip by sip.

Patients who do not need to lose weight should take 2–3 dl of almond milk three times a day after the fresh juice. For their preparation, see the recipe section.

In any case, you may and should additionally drink as much tea as you like. Goldenrod tea and stinging nettle tea support the excretion of urine and accompanying metabolic waste products. Bitter teas promote excretion via the liver and gallbladder. At the end of the first juice day, you will usually experience a flood of urine, connected to a significant, healthful weight loss as an expression of the reduction in swelling of the soft connective tissue and its basic substance.

On the 7th day at the latest, you will generally perceive a clear sense of well-being, which will give way to a second, usually weaker and fast-passing healing crisis on day 10.

After each period on the raw juice regime, you can move on to the stage-II diet. If the juice regime took less than three days, we recommend weekly repetition alternating with stage II. Working persons feel powerful and awake from this procedure, so that they can perform this regime in a weekly rhythm, if necessary for weeks or months.

Menu plan for the stage-I diet
It is very important that you observe the general suggestions for this raw-juice regime stage to enjoy the full healing effect.

Full Juice Day
In the morning 2 × 200 g fruit juice
200 g almond milk

For lunch   2 × 200 g fruit juice
             200 g almond milk
             200 g vegetable juice

In the evening as in the morning

No later
than around
8:00 p.m.   as desired 200 g
             fruit or vegetable juice

Almond milk contains very valuable unsaturated almond oil. In cases of insufficient liver function, oil cannot be digested and must be replaced by fruit and vegetable juices.

Serve fruit and vegetable juices immediately after pressing. Any waiting reduces their value.

Suggestions for fruit and vegetable juices (unmixed and tasty mixtures) and the recipe for almond milk or optional boiled gruel as an addition to the juices can be found in the recipe section.

Diet Stage II

This regime stage contains the whole rich range of raw food. The meals should be started with fresh juices or at least with fruits if possible. Three meals are suitable. If you feel hungry in between, you can easily have a little fruit or fresh juice. Since this diet is easy on the organism, you will not experience the "specific dynamic" redundant-heat effect from degradation of useless food. The regime therefore has a cooling effect. There may be a temporary reduction of the body's own heat that will be replaced by a spontaneous periodic warming of the organism by a kind of switching reaction in the metabolism and hormone system. If you feel cold during the raw-food diet you can prepare warm soup from freshly steamed vegetables as described in the recipe section. If tasty vegetables such as savoy cabbage, tomatoes and onion are used, salting is not necessary.

The raw vegetables may be prepared with a fine salad dressing that should not contain any animal products and as little salt as possible. Suitable recipes are continued in this book as well.

If you do not need to lose weight, we recommend eating almonds and unroasted nuts of many different kinds as well as sunflower and pumpkin seeds. During your first time at this stage, you will often feel periodic craving for salt that can be easily satisfied with the vegetable soup. If you have a strong craving for bread and baked things, you may nibble almonds. Cravings for sweets can be countered by fruits and possibly dried fruits. Such cravings usually all disappear entirely after a week or two, however, and will be replaced by a much more discriminating taste.

You can eat quite a bit when invited out to dinner at this diet stage, and the occasional exception will usually be well tolerated if you can dispense with fatty and animal products.

The stage-II diet can be used for many months if necessary without causing any deficit of any nutrient. It is complete and high-quality and leads to a special well-being and great mental and physical ability to cope well.

Menu plan for the stage-II diet

Breakfast and dinner remain the same for all days. Variety is added by the fruit used according to season (one type alone or tasty mixes). For this diet stage, Bircher muesli is prepared according to the original recipe with orange juice; see recipe section. In the evening, you can replace the ground nuts with almond milk (approx. 2 dl) and the fruits with fruit juice (approx. 2 dl). These juices must be drunk slowly in sips and well insalivated.

120–200 g	Birchermuesli
10 g	ground almonds or hazelnuts fruits as desired
1 cup	rosehip tea

Lunch

100–150 g	fruits or
50–100 g	cool fruit soup
50–100 g	romaine lettuce
100–150 g	raw-vegetable platter
20 g	nuts of all kinds (not salted or roasted)
200 g	optional 1 glass of unfermented apple or grape juice

As a suggestion, we provide you with seven examples each of raw-food compositions for the four seasons. Let your imagination and preferences inspire you as well. Place special value on raw bulb, root and leaf vegetables. Spice your dressings for raw food preferably with caraway or rosemary, since both are strongly detoxifying for the liver. Always start with seasonal fruit or iced fruit soup.

Spring:

1st day	radishes – fennel – head lettuce
2nd day	carrots – tomatoes – cress
3rd day	carrots – chicory – rocket
4th day	radish – lettuce – cress
5th day	red beet – dandelion – head lettuce
6th day	broccoli – spinach – cress
7th day	kohlrabi – tomatoes – head lettuce

Summer:

1st day	tomatoes – head lettuce – radish
2nd day	courgettes – rocket – carrots
3rd day	broccoli – radishes – head lettuce
4th day	kohlrabi – cress – head lettuce
5th day	stalk celery – lettuce – head lettuce
6th day	tomatoes filled with cauliflower – head lettuce
7th day	carrots – cucumbers – rocket

Autumn:

1st day	carrots – tomatoes – endives
2nd day	black salsify – spinach – head lettuce
3rd day	red beet – peperoni – head lettuce
4th day	broccoli – lamb's lettuce – endives
5th day	carrots – courgettes – cress
6th day	radish – tomatoes – head lettuce
7th day	radishes – cucumber – rocket

Winter:

1st day	black salsify – red cabbage – endives
2nd day	white cabbage – radicchio – head lettuce
3rd day	carrots – bell pepper – head lettuce
4th day	red beet – sauerkraut – endives
5th day	broccoli – spinach – lamb's lettuce
6th day	tomatoes – chicory – rocket
7th day	carrots – savoy cabbage – endives

The Stage-III Diet

This corresponds to an almost fat-free standard vegetarian regime with only carefully selected fat-free dairy products, basically some lean quark.

All recipes not marked with an asterisk are suitable for this stage. Patients who have experienced digestion problems such as flatulence and badly digested, badly formed stool while eating considerable amounts of bread and other flour-based foods, probably suffer from a wheat incompatibility. They should inform their doctor and only eat wheat in very small amounts, if at all, until their wheat allergy is healed. However, observe that this is usually connected to a milk allergy, which should be professionally diagnosed. Blood tests are not always reliable. Careful anamnesis and observation and possibly a test diet are more helpful. If food incompatibilities are not observed, there will be a deterioration once you move from stage II to stage III. The allergy will impair the intestinal environment so that the entero-hepatic circuit is not restored. In this case, individual adjustment of the stage-III diet by your doctor is required.

The stage-III diet is used once all liver symptoms have disappeared. It has proven beneficial to use stage II again for one or two weeks now and then to prevent recurrences. Interim juice days are also helpful, and should be followed by 3–4 days at stage II before returning to stage III.

Menu plan for 1 week for the stage-III diet

*In case of wheat allergy, replace wheat wholemeal or crisp bread with spelt or rye or barley.

The daily proportion of raw food should be 70 %.

All cooked dishes are made entirely without fat, the vegetables are steamed soft or crisp in fat-free vegetable bouillon and flavoured with herbs (as fresh as possible). E.g. smooth parsley and chives have lots of taste and are great for flavouring soups, which should also made only with fat-free vegetable bouillon. Fresh thyme and rosemary, basil, oregano, chervil etc. will add lots of taste to the dishes. A rather more eastern touch is added to the vegetables or soups by Ayurveda spices.

We recommend 1 small cup of bitter tea, ½ hour before lunch, and 1 cup of peppermint tea or horseradish juice around 4 p.m.

Breakfast
This meal is the same for all days:
grated apple with lemon and honey
or Bircher muesli with butter milk and honey wholegrain bread*
or crisp bread* with honey herbal tea or butter milk

1st day

Lunch
fruits of all kinds
raw vegetables, possibly whole and unchopped:
1 carrot, 1 tomato, some lettuce leaves whole or cut and chopped with a little lemon juice and lean yoghurt and herbs
vegetable bouillon
fennel with chives or parsley
rice with a little miso

Dinner
Grapefruit with honey
wholegrain bread* with honey
oat soup
rosehip tea with honey or butter milk

2nd day

Lunch
fruits
raw vegetables: celery root (celeriac) and whole, natural fennel, lamb's lettuce with lemon juice and herbs
spinach
caraway potatoes
apples baked in the oven with raisins, grapes and a little honey

Dinner
grated apples and bananas with lemon and honey
dried fruit (dates, figs, wine berries)
wholegrain bread* or crisp bread* with tomato
rosehip or herbal tea

3rd day
Lunch
fruits
raw vegetables: broccoli florets and tomato, prepared on head-lettuce leaves with lemon juice and herbs
barley gruel soup
celery root (celeriac)
polenta with herbs

Dinner
fruit salad with lemon and honey
rice with half-steamed tomatoes
herbal tea

4th day
Lunch
fruits
raw vegetables: carrot or horseradish juice, cucumber, cress
black salsify
potato puree

Dinner
fruits and dried fruit
potato soup with plenty of herbs
wholegrain bread*
rosehip tea

5th day
Lunch
fruits
raw vegetables: horseradish or horseradish juice, stalk celery, head lettuce, spinach soup
fresh romaine lettuce
wholegrain pasta with tomato sauce of pureed tomatoes with herbs

Dinner
fruit juice
potatoes boiled in their skins
cucumber salad or cooked carrot salad with lemon and herbs

6th day
Lunch
fruits
raw vegetables: red beet or red beet juice, courgettes and spinach leaves, artichokes with vinaigrette without oil, potato puree with carrot sauce (pureed carrots with fat-free bouillon)
applesauce

Dinner
1 grapefruit eaten with a spoon
rice and vegetable soup
crisp bread* with honey
herbal tea or butter milk

7th day
Lunch
fruits
raw vegetables: radish, tomatoes, head lettuce leaves
vegetable bouillon
stewed tomatoes
Japanese rice

Dinner
fruit salad with lemon and honey
baked potatoes
cooked red beet salad with lemon
steamed spinach with lemon
herbal tea or butter milk

The Stage-IV Diet

This is a low-fat, liver-protecting diet that therefore prevents relapses of enterohepatic crises. Continue eating in this manner after healing. This diet will also prevent most other chronic diseases such as cancer, cardiovascular diseases, rheumatism etc. Even Ayurveda, the medical healing art of Ancient India, assumed that this kind of nutrition would lead to a life expectancy of a hundred years with wonderful mental and physical health.

Put in periods at stage II now and then, e.g. for one week per month or more. Always go from stage II to stage IV via stage III.

Menu plan for 1 week for the stage-IV diet
*In case of wheat allergy, replace wheat wholemeal or crisp bread with spelt or rye or barley.

The daily proportion of raw food should be 60–70 %.

Breakfast is the same for all days:

Bircher muesli or fruits or fruit juice
nuts, whole or ground
wholegrain bread* or crisp bread* with max. 10 g premium butter or nut spread
rosehip tea or herbal tea

Dinner variations
Bircher muesli or fruits or raw fruit salad or ½ grapefruit with a soup or baked potatoes with lean quark with herbs and salad or sandwiches and salad or a rice or pasta dish with salad

Lunch variations

1st day
fruits, dried fruit
raw vegetables: carrots, endives, head lettuce
vegetable broth with bread cubes
black salsify, steamed potatoes with tomato

2nd day
fruits, dried fruit
raw vegetables: red beet, cucumbers, cress
stuffed tomatoes
lemon cream

3rd day
fruits
raw vegetables: celery root (celeriac), tomatoes, lamb's lettuce
semolina soup
chopped cabbage
caraway potatoes

4th day
fruits
raw vegetables: black salsify, spinach, endives
carrots in sauce
polenta
apple compote

5th day
fruits
raw vegetables: horseradish, courgettes, head lettuce
vegetable soup
cabbage stalks steamed in vegetable bouillon
Lyonnaise potatoes

6th day
fruits
raw vegetables: cauliflower, cress, head lettuce
chervil soup
spinach
pasta with tomato sauce

7th day
fruits
raw vegetables: tomatoes stuffed with celery root (celeriac) salad, head lettuce
courgettes
mashed potato
stuffed apples

Small substitution table for animal products that must be left out in the stage-III diet

Instead of butter
Health-food store vegetable margarine, unhardened (ensure that it does not contain any milk protein according to the ingredients list on the package), as bread spread; health-food store vegetable fat for steaming and baking; nut spread for melting

The health-food store will offer various types of nut spread (almond spread, cashew spread, mixed spread of several nuts) that are not only suitable for raw use but also – stirred smooth with a little water – can be heated briefly and put on vegetables or potatoes. Sesame paste is also good for this.

Instead of cream
Soy cream from the health-food store for sauces and cooked dishes; it cannot be beaten, however. Almond cream of almond puree, with water and a little sea salt or honey (depending on use), whipped creamy with a whisk

Instead of milk
Milk is a bit harder to replace. It can often (e.g. in soups) just be left out and replaced with an equivalent amount of water. Depending on recipe and in drinks, almond milk, soy and sesame milk, pine nut milk, rice milk and coconut milk can be used (see recipes).

Instead of yoghurt
Yoghurt is hard to replace as well. The health-food store will sell soy yoghurt, but usually sweetened! The recipes for Bircher muesli have enough great versions without yoghurt, however, and nuts and fresh fruits or dried fruit, and possibly a piece of rye or spelt crispbread with vegetable margarine make a great snack.

Instead of eggs
Arrowroot flour or cornflour or potato flour for binding. Tofu: 50 g tofu per 1 egg, pureed

Instead of mayonnaise
Almond mayonnaise or mayonnaise of soy wholegrain flour without added wheat (see recipes)

Instead of cheese and quark
Ground cheese in vegetables, soups, pasta products etc. is just left out. Cheese and quark for sandwiches are replaced by pure plant spreads and additions to salads by ready-made tofu-burgers, etc. (observe in the ingredients list that no milk or egg white, wheat and mushroom parts are contained).

Instead of wheat
All other cereal types can be used for cereal dishes. In bread, wheat flour is unfortunately mixed in rye or barley or spelt breads as well, so ask specifically and study the ingredients list of crisp breads.

The Recipes

During the strict diet (stages I and II), use only those recipes that are not marked with an asterisk (*); the mild food stages can use all recipes. If one or another ingredient is marked with an asterisk (*), it should be left out for the strict diet (levels I and II).

Juices

Juices are "raw fruits and vegetables" in a mechanically refined form, used as additional special enrichment and for patients with gastrointestinal diseases, when coarse food (cellulose) is not permitted. Whole raw vegetables are always higher in quality and cannot be replaced by juice permanently. The disintegration of the plant cells in the juice press, however, releases a higher energy potential that is very important for inducing healing via the basic system. A healing regime therefore should always be started with fresh juices, and should continue to contain them.

For preparation of juices, the raw vegetables are cleaned thoroughly (see chapter raw vegetables), pressed with a hand press or an electrical centrifugal juicer and served immediately. Any resting time reduces their value.

Fruit juices
a) Unmixed fruit juices:
  orange, tangerine, grapefruit, apple, pear, grape, strawberry, blueberry, currant, cassis, raspberry, peach, apricot, plum, mango, Japanese persimmon, kiwi

b) Mixed fruit juices, e.g.:
  orange, tangerine, grapefruit, Japanese persimmon or berry juice with apple juice or berry juice with peach, apricot or plum juice or beaten bananas with orange, berry, peach, mango or apricot juice

Additions as desired or required: lemon juice, honey, maple syrup, fruit concentrate, cream*, yoghurt*, almond milk*.

Vegetable Juices
Drunk freshly, they have a high mineral and vitamin content. Each juice has its own special value.

a) Unmixed vegetable juices:
  tomato, carrot, red beet, radish, cabbage, celery root (celeriac), and all leaf, bulb and root vegetable; stinging nettle, sorrel and dandelion juice for springtime blood-cleansing treatment
b) Mixed vegetable juices:
  carrot, tomato, and spinach in equal proportions (very tasty)
  tomato and carrot
  tomato and spinach

Other mixes (and cocktails) can be combined as desired.

For variety, add sorrel, stinging nettle, chives, parsley, onions, celery root (celeriac) leaves or bulbs and other herbs.

Additions per glass (1½–2 dl): 1 teaspoon almond puree or 1 tablespoon buttermilk, some lemon juice, or some fruit concentrate (optional).

c) Potato juice:
   Prepare well-cleaned, peeled potatoes (no unripe, green or sprouted ones) like carrot juice. Not flavourful, but relieves cramps and is particularly effective for heartburn and for stomach and duodenal ulcers.

Gruel to Go with Juices
The gruel is added to raw juices at a proportion of ⅓; it neutralises the sharpness of the fruit or vegetable flavour. The daily ration can be prepared once a day and kept in a thermos bottle until use.

a) Rice or barley gruel:
   Stir 1 heaped teaspoon rice or barley wholemeal flour with 2 dl cold water and boil for 5 min., stirring constantly. Let cool.
b) Flax seed gruel:
   Wash 1 tablespoon flax seeds, boil in 2 dl water for 10 min., strain and let cool.

Healthful Teas

Use whole leaves for teas if possible, since the essential oils are lost when the leaves are chopped more finely (sachet form). Bitter and flatulence teas are drunk unsweetened, while other teas can have some honey and/or diluted lemon juice added.

Bitter tea
Wormwood
Centaurium
Cnicus
Mix in equal parts, boil slightly and steep for 5 min.
For lack of appetite, drink 2–3 tablespoons ½ hour before meals (mildly cholagogic).
Sensitive persons should use only centaurium.

Wormwood tea
Boil slightly and steep for 5 min.
Strong bitter tea, strongly cholagogic, gastric-juice stimulating.
Drink in sips during the day.

Flatulence tea
Caraway
Fennel
Aniseed
Mix in equal parts, boil slightly and steep for 20 min.
Have 1 cup after meals against flatulence.

Chamomile tea
Only boil slightly.
Drink for stomach pain.
Cleansing effect and calming on the gastrointestinal tract.
For enemas and rinsing.

Peppermint tea
Only boil slightly.
Calming, cholagogic.

Vervain tea
Only boil slightly.
Calming, mucous reducing, cholagogic; very popular tea in France.

Lemon-balm tea
Only boil slightly.
Very calming, good before sleeping.

Lemon-peel tea
Thinly cut off the peel of 1 untreated lemon, boil for approx. 5 min. with ½ l water, let steep for 10 min. and strain.
Calming.

Orange-blossom tea
Boil 2–3 blossoms for 2–3 min., let steep and strain. Sweeten with honey.
Calming; drink before sleeping.

Flax seed tea
Boil 1 tablespoon flax seeds in ½ l water for 7–10 min. and let steep.
Mucous reducing, mildly laxative.

Lady's-mantle tea
Briefly boil 2 tablespoons of leaves in ½ l water, steep for 10 min.
Prevents gynaecological problems.

Alpine lady's-mantle tea
Like lady's-mantle tea.

Solidago tea
(golden rod, baneberry)
Boil 1 tablespoon solidago in ½ l water for 1 min., steep for 10 min.
For dropsy, bladder and kidney infections; water expelling.
2–3 cups per day.

Bearberry leaf tea
Briefly boil 1½ tablespoons bearberry leaves in 5 dl water for 5 min., steep for 10 min., strain.
For bladder infections.

Lavender tea
Briefly boil 1 teaspoon lavender leaves, steep a bit.
Calming, harmonising, anti-inflammatory, for sleeplessness.

Rosehip tea
Soak 2–3 tablespoons rosehip seeds and peels in 1 ½ l water for 12 hours, then slightly boil for ½–¾ hours, strain. The rest of the boiled rosehips can be boiled again with fresh ones on the next day.
Slightly cholagogic and water-expelling.

Birchermuesli

All recipes are only calculated for 1 person.

The original apple muesli as invented by Dr Bircher and used with his patients successfully thousands of times has remained the best food for the regime according to our long experience.

Sweet-tart, juicy applies with white flesh are best for the muesli, e.g. Klar apples, Gravenstein, Sauergrauech, Menznauer Jäger, Jonathan, Ontario, Rubinette, Glockenäpfel, Braeburn, Champagner-Reinetten, Cox's Orange.

The flavour of drier apple types with a weaker taste can be enriched with a little freshly ground peel of untreated oranges or lemons or with orange juice or a little rosehip paste or freshly ground ginger.

Birchermuesli with yoghurt or sour or buttermilk*
1 tablespoon (8 g) oat flakes
3 tablespoon water
2 tablespoon Bifidus-yoghurt or Bifidus sour or buttermilk
1 teaspoon honey
200 g apples
1 tablespoon hazelnuts or almonds, ground

Soak the oat flakes for 12 hours (for breakfast overnight). Mix the oat flakes with the yoghurt or sour milk and honey into a smooth sauce. Remove stems and calyxes from the washed apples and grate them directly into the sauce. Stir several times to keep the muesli pleasantly white. Spread the nuts on it and serve at once. Never let it rest.

Versions: Replace oat flakes with wheat, rice, barley, rye, semolina, buckwheat or soy flakes, or optionally mix them with yeast flakes (enriching with vitamin B).

Different version: Mix 1 teaspoon soaked oat flakes with 1 teaspoon cereal grains (soak in water for 24 hours, then empty onto a screen and rinse cold, wholly, chopped or pureed).

Birchermuesli with almond or sesame puree*
1 tablespoon (8 g) oat flakes
3 tablespoons water

½ tablespoon lemon juice
1 tablespoon almond or sesame puree
1 tablespoon honey
3 tablespoons water
200 g apples
1 tablespoon hazelnuts or almonds, ground

Soak the oat flakes for 12 hours. Stir lemon juice, puree, honey and water into a creamy sauce with a whisk, add oat flakes and apples (as described in the basic recipe). Sprinkle with nuts, serve at once.

Birchermuesli with orange juice
1 tablespoon (8 g) fine oat flakes
3 tablespoons water
1 tablespoon lemon juice
½ orange, squeezed
200 g apples
1 tablespoon hazelnuts or almonds, ground
Prepared like basic recipe.

Birchermuesli with berries or stone fruit
(particularly rich in vitamin C)
Prepare an almond or sesame* puree sauce or yoghurt* sauce. Finish by adding:
150–200 g strawberries or raspberries, blueberries, currants or blackberries, and mash slightly with a fork
or
150–200 g plums, peaches or apricots, pitted and ground through the chopper or cut finely with a knife. Avoid plums and apricots for patients with gastrointestinal problems.

Birchermuesli with various fruits
The following combinations are particularly tasty:
strawberries and raspberries
strawberries, raspberries and currants
strawberries and apples
blackberries and apples
apples with finely cut orange and tangerine pieces
apples and bananas
apples and peaches

sauce: almond puree or sesame* puree sauce or yoghurt* sauce
Only use fresh fruits, never use canned fruits (fruit salad, etc.!).

Birchermuesli with dried fruits
If you have no fresh fruits on hand, you can also make the muesli with dried fruits (apples, apricots, plums, pears). One hundred grams of dried fruits are washed, soaked in cold water for 12 hours and ground through the chopper. Mix with almond puree or sesame* puree sauce or yoghurt* sauce. For dried fruits, always look for good quality without preservatives or bleach; otherwise, gastrointestinal problems may occur.

Birchermuesli with condensed milk*
If you do not have almond or sesame puree or fresh yoghurt on hand, you can also make the muesli with condensed milk according to the original recipe, but only from Diet Stage III, as condensed milk is usually sugared.

Sprouted cereal grains
These are particularly high in the vitamin E and B group, and generally have a strengthening effect.

1st day, evening: wash the grains in a screen under running water and put them in a bowl. Cover with water and keep at room temperature, close to the oven.

2nd day, morning: rinse off and spread to dry on a flat plate at room temperature, close to the oven. The same evening, put them back in the bowl and cover with water. Keep at room temperature, close to the oven.

3rd day, morning: rinse off and spread to dry on the plate. Evening: put the grains back in the bowl and cover with water. Keep at room temperature, close to the oven.

On the 4th day, the grains should have developed sprouts of 1–2 cm and are ready to eat.

The preparation of sprouted cereal grains is easier in the practical sprouting devices that are available in different sizes.

Raw vegetables and Salads

Observe three considerations when preparing raw vegetables and salads:

1. Freshness and quality
For the liver diet (as well as for any other diet and for full everyday nutrition), use only sun-ripened, organically grown vegetables and salads. They are not only best for health but also have the best taste. Today, the offer from organically run operations is very large, and organically grown vegetables are available even in supermarkets. Of course it is particularly good to use vegetables and salads from your own garden. Herbs and tomatoes can be grown even on the balcony.

Chose young, tender leafy lettuces and root vegetables, not blanched, without any wilted leaves or rotting stalks. For a healing regime it is particularly important to use only entirely fresh and high-quality plants.

Prepare raw vegetables right before eating them and mix them with the dressing immediately. Letting them stand in the air will markedly reduce the vitamin content of the chopped vegetables and salads.

2. Cleaning well
Biologically grown vegetables without manure fertilisation contain no worm eggs. Nevertheless, all fresh plants must be cleaned thoroughly and carefully. Observe that water-soluble substances such as Vitamin C, vitamins of the B-group and minerals are leached out in water.

3. Harmonious composition
Every salad dish should contain the three aspects: root-fruit-leaf. Green leafy lettuce in particular is always part of a healing regime. In the dressings, variety is desirable for different ingredients of the raw food.

A beautifully assembled salad dish in pleasing colours will be enjoyed by the eye as well as the palate and will stimulate the appetite.

Small garnishes of herbs, radishes, young carrots or olives make the raw vegetable dish even more colourful and festive. The number three should not be exceeded per meal for everyday use. Too much variety may impair digestion.

Cleaning the leafy vegetables
For head lettuce, endives, romaine lettuce, iceberg lettuce and similar green leaf lettuces, cabbage and red cabbage, etc. take apart the leaves and clean them individually and carefully under running water. Rinse several times and spin until dry.

Small-leaved salads such as lamb's lettuce and cut lettuce, spinach, dandelion, cress, rocket, cicorino and Brussels sprouts get rinsed repeatedly in small portions and any hard stalks are removed.

Halve chicory, remove outer leaves and rinse well.

Cleaning the root vegetables
Celery, carrots, horseradish, radish, red beet, kohlrabi, black salsify: clean with a brush under running water, peel and immediately grate or plane into the finished sauce; mix well to keep the vegetables from losing their fresh colour.

Cleaning of vegetable fruits
Wash tomatoes and cut them into wedges or slices. Peel cucumbers and cut them

small or grate them. Biologically grown young cucumbers do not need to be peeled.

Use only young, tender courgettes for salads, wash them well, do not peel them, and cut them into rings or rods.

Green and yellow peperoni (bell pepper) is less hot than the red variety. Wash, halve, remove seeds and cut small. Unfortunately, almost all peperoni today are from hydroponic production.

Take apart cauliflower and broccoli into smaller bits, and prepare and clean thoroughly under running water. Wash stalk celery, peel it, and cut away hard parts.

Halve leeks and fennel, prepare and wash under the tap set to shower.

Salad dressings

In the acute stage of hepatitis, the small portions of salads that are permitted after the first juice days must be eaten entirely without dressings. Alternate the herbs often – this will avoid boredom! Today, you can purchase even herbs other than parsley and chives in good quality almost all year round.

Oil dressing*
1 tablespoon oil* (rapeseed, sunflower or olive oil from first cold pressing, thistle oil, walnut oil)
1 teaspoon lemon juice or organic fruit vinegar
optional garlic, pressed*
1 teaspoon fresh or 1 knife tip of dried herbs

Mix all ingredients and whisk the sauce until creamy. The sauce also becomes very tasty with a splash of soy sauce or Kelpamare.
This classic salad dressing is suited to all green salads (head lettuce, romaine lettuce, cress, etc.) and fruit salads (tomatoes, cucumbers etc.)

Quark sauce
1 tablespoon lean quark
3 tablespoons butter milk
½ teaspoon lemon juice
fresh, finely chopped herbs

Mix all ingredients well with a whisk. This dressing goes particularly well with root vegetables (carrots, celery root (celeriac), radishes etc.)

Yoghurt dressing
2–3 tablespoons yoghurt
some drops of lemon juice (optional)
optional onions, grated*
garlic, pressed*
1 teaspoon fresh or 1 knife tip of dried herbs

Mix all ingredients well with a whisk. A refreshing dressing with cress or spinach, with fruit salads (tomatoes, cucumbers) and with root vegetables (kohlrabi, horseradish, radishes)

Cream dressing*
2 tablespoons sour cream*
1 teaspoon lean quark
1 teaspoon lemon juice
very little pepper
1 teaspoon fresh or 1 knife tip of dried herbs

Mix all ingredients well with a whisk. This dressing suits almost all root and fruit salads. For diversity, you may replace lemon juice with orange juice, to give the raw food a new flavour. With celery root (celeriac), red beet and chicory salad, you can add a little freshly ground horseradish to this sauce for a very exciting taste.

Lemon dressing*
2 tablespoons freshly pressed lemon juice
1 tablespoon agave syrup (Allos)

1 teaspoon olive oil
a little grated onion
1 teaspoon salad herbs mixture or Ysop
Mix all ingredients well.

This dressing suits all salads, particularly dark green leafy salads. In spring, add a few daisies to the green salad – they are very rich in nutrients and look pretty.

Orange dressing
1 small lemon
2 large oranges
1 tablespoon freshly ground coriander
1 piece fresh ginger
(for 2 dl sauce)

Press oranges and lemon and mix well; add coriander and finely ground ginger. If you like your dressing slightly sweet (particularly good with carrots or red beet), add 1 teaspoon thick agave juice (Allos). The root vegetables should be marinated in the dressing for at least 3 hours. Before serving, you can drip a very small amount of olive oil on the salad.

Garlic dressing*
1 garlic clove
(in spring, 2 wild-onion leaves)
2 tablespoons thistle or sunflower oil*
1 tablespoon apple vinegar
1 tablespoon unrefined sugar (Panela, Succanat)

Put the sugar in the vinegar overnight to dissolve it completely. Mix oil and vinegar well with a whisk; add the pressed garlic clove or finely cut wild-onion leaves. This dressing tastes great with vegetable-blossom salads such as broccoli, cauliflower or romanesco.

Peppermint dressing
2 tablespoons freshly pressed lemon juice
1 tablespoon honey or agave syrup
1 tablespoon olive oil* (optional)
lots of fresh peppermint leaves

Mix liquid ingredients well with the whisk. Cut the peppermint leaves finely and mix them in as well.
This scented, green dressing goes wonderfully with sugar peas, but also with finely cut romaine lettuce.

Nut dressing*
2 tablespoons sour cream*
1 tablespoon hazelnut or almond paste*
1 teaspoon lemon juice
A little honey
1 pinch of ginger
1 tablespoon coarsely chopped walnuts, hazelnuts or almonds

Mix all ingredients well with the whisk. A pretty sauce for root vegetables that also goes well with Belgian endive cut into fine slices. For variety, you may add a little finely cut apple.

Almond- or sesame-puree dressing*
1 tablespoon almond- or sesame puree*
3 tablespoons water
1 teaspoon lemon juice
garlic, pressed (optional)
1 teaspoon fresh or 1 knife tip of dried herbs

Slowly stir sesame or almond puree with water until smooth, then add the other ingredients.
This very tasty sauce goes very well with root vegetables.

Mayonnaise with wholegrain soy flour instead of egg*
Mayonnaise – even without egg, and even if "stretched" with yoghurt – remains an enjoyment that liver patients must only permit themselves in exceptions and in small portions (only at stage IV, of course), since the oil cannot be replaced.

(for 6–8 portions)
2 tablespoons wholegrain soy flour
6 tablespoons water
2 dl oil*

Mix wholegrain soy flour and water into a smooth mass, and slowly add oil under constant stirring with the whisk.
The mayonnaise can be kept in the fridge for a few days.
For 1 portion, you need:

1 tablespoon mayonnaise
1 teaspoon lemon juice
mustard (optional)
1 teaspon fresh or 1 knife tip of dried herbs

Mix all ingredients well. Mayonnaise is a popular dressing with many fruit salads and root vegetables.

Sauerkraut salad*
Sauerkraut is a particularly valuable raw vegetable, especially in winter. It is more easily digestible raw than cooked and has a gallbladder-purging and disinfecting effect. An addition of cut small raw sauerkraut can improve taste and tolerability considerably. For a salad, sauerkraut is loosened up and cut small, mixed with a few caraway seeds or ground caraway, 3 – 4 chopped juniper berries, chopped onion and an apple cut into small strips or diced small fresh pineapple. Choose oil dressing* or mayonnaise of wholegrain soy flour* as a dressing. This salad goes particularly well with corn salad and a raw root vegetable.

Milk Types

All milk types listed here (apart from soy milk and almond milk) may only be consumed in the stage-IV diet.

Almond milk
This food provides vegetable protein and oil, and is rich in valuable unsaturated vegetable oils.
Stimulates mucous production and soothes.

1 tablespoon almond puree
1½ teaspoons honey
1½ dl water and ½ dl fruit juice (causes slight thickening)

Mix almond puree and honey with the whisk and add water by droplets. Add fruit juice last.

Fresh almond milk
Particularly easy to digest

1½ tablespoons almonds, peeled (no bitter ones!)
1 teaspoons honey
1½ dl water

Mix almonds, honey and water in the mixer, strain if necessary.

Pine nut milk
Very rich in easily digestible vegetable oils and protein that protects the metabolism.

1½ tablespoons pine nuts, washed
1 teaspoon honey
1½ dl water

Prepare like almond milk.

Sesame milk
2 dl water (cold or warm)
1 level tablespoon sesame puree
1 teaspoon lemon juice
1 teaspoon honey

Mix sesame puree and honey with the whisk and add the water by the drop. Finally add the lemon juice.

Sesame cream
Like sesame milk, but with less water added; replaces cream in cooked dishes and desserts.

Sesame frappé/milkshake
Like sesame milk or sesame cream, with addition of fruit juice or fruit concentrates.

Soy milk
1 cup soy beans
7 cups of water
1 tablespoon fruit sugar
water

Wash and dry soy beans and grind them in an almond mill. Soak for 2 hours, then boil in the soaking water for 20 min., stirring constantly. Strain. Add water until the viscosity of cows' milk is reached. Add fruit sugar and let cool. Soy milk is sold in tetra packs in the health-food store.

Butter, plant and vegetable fats and oils Light cooking and steaming

The Bircher kitchen uses only cold-pressed oils, almond and other nut spreads for raw food; cooked food may also be prepared using small amounts of fresh butter and vegetable fats. Vegetable oils generally should not be heated, since heating may turn the highly unsaturated fatty acids into dangerous radicals. The only exception is olive oil with a very high share of simply unsaturated fatty acids. It may also be used for hot cuisine.

Fresh butter
In the amounts named, it may be used to enrich dishes for liver-gallbladder patients from the stage-IV diet onwards.

Health-food store vegetable margarine and health-food store food fats
(in Switzerland, e.g. Nussella, Becel, Olima, in Germany Vitaquell, Eden) are vegetable-fat emulsions of naturally firm, i.e. unhardened fats such as coconut oil or palm-seed oil with their considerable content of liquid oils and seed oils, too, in particular sunflower or olive oil.

Nut spread and almond puree
These preparations have a very fine, nut-like flavour. They can be used variously as bland food or to replace fresh butter or vegetable margarine with vegetables, potatoes, rice, and pasta products.

Cold-pressed sunflower oil, corn oil, thistle oil, flax seed oil, cold-pressed olive oil
Organic and carefully treated, rich in highly unsaturated fatty acids, these fats are more easily digestible for most people than heated butter. However, as mentioned, the vegetable oils should not be heated, since heating may produce dangerous radicals (exception: olive oil). Flax seed oil has a very distinctive flavour and is particularly recommended as a treatment for liver patients: 2×2 tablespoons per day; do not leave the oil in an open container, but keep it tightly closed in the fridge. The addition of lemon juice protects against oxidation.

Light cooking and steaming
Today, hardly any housewife or working woman will want to do without her pressure cooker. This appliance is time-saving and far more healthful than other methods. Who would want to forgo these advantages?

The pressure cooker works especially well for soups, and is useful for almost every other recipe. It reduces cooking time by $\frac{1}{3}$ to $\frac{1}{4}$. Many vegetable and potato recipes also can be steamed gently and very quickly in the pressure cooker, resulting in dishes that retain their colour, taste, vitamins and nutrients. By the way, the cooking time of vegetables (except potatoes) can be reduced as desired even with conventional steaming if you like your vegetables crunchier, "al dente". For cereal dishes, we recommend using the steamer for grains with long cooking times (e.g. coarse corn), but not for pasta products.

Soups

The recipes are calculated for 1–2 persons.

The following soup and vegetable recipes use a lot of vegetable broth. In a small household, it will not pay of to make fresh vegetable broth every day. Instead, you may use ordinary water and spice with health-food store yeast extract (liquid or paste) or vegetarian salt-free vegetable bouillon cubes. The health-food store yeast extracts are very rich in vitamin B and in important glutathione and lecithin. Caution: yeast extract is allowed as a cover name for the harmful glutamate, so make sure when buying! Cream* enriches soups and vegetables, but you can usually use milk instead.

In case of wheat allergy, the wholegrain flour in the recipes should be replaced by rice, millet or oat flour.

Vegetable broth
As the only exception, this recipe is calculated for 4 persons

1 tablespoon health-food store vegetable fat*
1 onion
2 carrots
1 small stalk of celery (150 g)
cabbage, Swiss chard leaves
1 leek stem
3–4 l water
½ bay leaf
1 pinch sea salt
lovage, basil or other herbs, dried or preferably fresh

Halve the onion, keeping the brown peel, and brown the cut area in the hot fat. Cut the vegetables small, add them and steam for at least 15 min. covered at low heat. Add water and cook for 2 hours at low heat. Season as desired.
For the stage-III diet (fat-free), let the vegetables steam without fat with the peel and onion also cut in small pieces and then continue for 15 min. with the addition of a little water. Continue as above.

Vegetable bouillon
3 dl vegetable broth
health-food store yeast extract (optional)
10 g nut spread* or health-food store vegetable fat*, parsley, chives, freshly chopped herbs

Prepare the vegetable broth according to the above recipe with nut spread* or vegetable fat* and herbs. Season with yeast extract or Kelpamare if desired.

Rice soup, clear
½ tablespoon health-food store vegetable fat*
some chopped onion
1 small carrot
some celery root (celeriac) and leek
1 tablespoon rice
6 dl vegetable broth
chives

Steam onion, finely cut vegetables and rice together. Add hot vegetable broth and cook for 15–20 minutes. Prepare with finely cut chives and vegetable fat*.

Rice soup, thickened*
½ tablespoon health-food store vegetable fat*
some celery root (celeriac)
1 small carrot
some leek
1 tablespoon rice
½ tablespoon wholegrain flour
6 dl vegetable broth or water
1 pinch sea salt
lovage, parsley, basil, marjoram
health-food store yeast extract
½ tablespoon sesame cream
chives

Steam the finely cut vegetables and rice in fat. Spread wholegrain flour on them, add the vegetable broth and cook for 30 minutes. Season with yeast extract and herbs. Put cream and finely cut chives in the soup bowl and pour the soup into it.

Herbal soup
1 tablespoon wholegrain flour
1 dl milk* or water
5 dl vegetable broth
1 tablespoon cream*
5 g butter* or vegetable margarine* or nut spread* (optional)
1 pinch of sea salt
lovage, basil, tarragon, marjoram, chives, optional nutmeg or caraway

Stir wholegrain flour into a little cold milk* or cold water and add to the boiling vegetable broth.
Cook for 15 minutes.
Season with the herbs; if permitted, add cream* or optional butter* or vegetable margarine* to the soup bowl, add the soup and whisk.

Oat cream soup
½ tablespoon health-food store vegetable fat*
2 tablespoons fine or coarse oat flakes
6 dl vegetable broth
some celery root (celeriac)
1 tablespoon sesame cream
1 pinch sea salt
Kelpamare, chives, optional nutmeg or caraway

Briefly steam oats flakes with or without vegetable fat. Add vegetable broth and celery root (celeriac). Slightly cook oat flakes for 10 minutes, coarse ones for at least 20 minutes, and season as desired. Put cream*, sea salt and chives in the soup bowl and add the pureed soup.

Oat groats soup
½ tablespoon health-food store vegetable fat*
2 tablespoons porridge
some onion, chopped
7 dl water or vegetable broth

1 dl milk*
some celery root (celeriac), diced
1 pinch of sea salt
1 tablespoon cream* (optional)
yeast extract, chives, parsley, marjoram or borage

Steam onion and groats with or without vegetable fat*. Add vegetable broth, milk* and celery root (celeriac) and cook for 45–60 minutes. Season as desired with health-food store yeast extract; Put cream*, sea salt and herbs in the soup bowl and pour the finished soup into it.

Semolina soup
1 tablespoon semolina
5 dl vegetable broth
1 tablespoon sesame cream
5 g fresh butter*, vegetable fat* or nut spread*
1 pinch of sea salt, soy sauce
nutmeg, optional caraway
lovage, basil, marjoram, parsley, chives

Stir semolina into the boiling vegetable broth, add soy sauce and caraway, and cook for ½ hour. Season as desired with sea salt and herbs. Put cream* and butter* or health-food store vegetable fat* or nut spread* in the soup bowl and pour the finished soup into it.

Tomato soup
½ tablespoon health-food store vegetable fat*
some onion, celery root (celeriac) and leek
1 small carrot
1 garlic clove
1 tomato
1 tablespoon wholegrain flour
6 dl vegetable broth
1 pinch of sea salt
some tomato puree (optional)
1 pinch of fruit sugar
rosemary, oregano
5 g butter* or vegetable margarine* or nut spread*
1 tablespoon sesame cream
chives

Steam vegetables cut small with or without vegetable fat*, then add the tomato. Sprinkle with wholegrain flour and pour the vegetable broth into the mixture. Cook for ½ hour, then strain. Add spices and optional tomato puree. Put butter* or health-food store vegetable fat* (or nut spread*) and cream* in the soup bowl and pour the finished soup into it. Sprinkle with finely cut chives. If desired, add 1 tablespoon rice to the soup or sprinkle with fat-free toasted bread cubes.

Summery tomato soup
4 ripe summer tomatoes
1 pinch of fruit sugar
1 pinch sea salt
¼ dl cream*

Cut the tomatoes into pieces, cook briefly, season and strain. Add cream* and serve the soup lukewarm or cold.

Various vegetable soups (carrots, spinach, broccoli)
½ tablespoon health-food store vegetable fat*
some chopped onion
1½ tablespoons wholegrain flour
1 pinch of sea salt
5 dl vegetable broth
1 dl milk*
1 tablespoon sesame cream*

Vegetables: 1 carrot, cut small, or 1 small cup of spinach, pureed or finely chopped, broccoli finely chopped (cook some florets separately and reserve them).

Steam onion and carrots or broccoli with or without vegetable fat*, sprinkle with wholegrain flour and steam them together slightly. Add vegetable broth and milk* and cook for 20–40 minutes. For the spinach soup, add the spinach last and do not cook longer. Pour the finished soup onto the cream* in the soup bowl. For the broccoli soup, add the reserved florets.

Seasoning: For the carrot soup, use celery greens or lovage, rosemary or marjoram, 1 teaspoon caraway.

For the spinach soup, use some peppermint leaves, parsley, chives, 1 pinch of nutmeg.

For the broccoli soup, use yeast extract, a little basil, parsley, chives, tarragon.

Chervil soup
½ tablespon health-food store vegetable fat*
some onion
1 medium-sized potato, chopped in cubes
½ tablespoon wholegrain flour
5 dl vegetable broth
1 pinch sea salt
1 tablespoon chervil, chopped
1 tablespoon cream*

Steam the onion slightly with or without vegetable fat*. Add potato, sprinkle with wholegrain flour and add vegetable broth and salt. Cook for ½ hour and strain. Put chervil and cream* in the soup bowl and pour the soup into it.

Potato soup
½ leek, cut into thin strips
½ carrot, cut into small disks
½ tablespoon wholegrain flour
5 dl vegetable broth
1 medium-sized potato, chopped into small pieces
1 pinch of sea salt
Miso
basil, marjoram
1 tablespoon cream*

Steam leek and carrot in a little vegetable broth. Sprinkle with wholegrain flour and add the vegetable broth. Add potato and cook until soft. Season. Put basil, marjoram and optional cream* in the soup bowl and pour the finished soup into it.

Minestrone
2 tablespoon leek
some onion, chopped
some celery root (celeriac) leaves
½ plateful red beet greens
7 dl water or vegetable broth
1 tablespoon lovage or thyme
½ garlic clove, pressed
basil, parsley, chives
1 pinch of sea salt
15 g pasta or rice
5 g butter* or health-food store vegetable fat* or nut spread*

Finely chop onion, leek, celery leaves and beet greens and steam them slowly. Add vegetable broth, season and cook for ½ hour. Add pasta products or rice and cook for 15–20 minutes. To enrich, add cream* or nut spread* or health-food store vegetable fat*.

Vegetables

Vegetables "nature", fat-free
When moving from the stage-II diet to stage III, sensitive patients will be offered vegetables "naturally": The vegetable is steamed until soft in a little fat-free vegetable broth, then chopped according to vegetable type and prepared with herbs. The following vegetables are particularly recommended for liver patients: romaine lettuce, chicory, fennel, carrots, celery, tomatoes, red beet, artichokes, broccoli. Spinach, endives, Swiss chard, stalk celery, peas, sugar peas, courgettes, peperoni, kohlrabi, cauliflower, Jerusalem artichoke and aubergines can be prepared in this way as well.

Spinach, chopped
¼ l vegetable broth
200 g spinach (remove thick stems)
¼ garlic clove, pressed
1 pinch of sea salt
peppermint leaves, sage
1 cup raw spinach
optional fresh butter* or health-food store vegetable fat* or olive oil*

Briefly boil spinach in the vegetable broth, drain, cut, chop or mix. Return spinach to the pan and heat. Add garlic, salt and herbs. Very finely chop or mix the raw spinach and add a little optional butter* or olive oil* before serving.

Spinach, whole leaves (and stems)
300 g spinach (remove thick stems, briefly boil the coarser winter spinach if required)
1 tablespoon pine nuts
1 tablespoon raisins (optional)
1 pinch of sea salt
peppermint leaves, sage, parsley
optional melted butter* or health-food store vegetable fat* or olive oil*

Steam spinach uncovered on low heat with very little water. Add pine nuts, spices and optional raisins and continue steaming briefly. Finally mix in some liquid butter* or olive oil* if desired.

Lettuce
1 head of lettuce
1 l water
some chopped onion
1 dl vegetable broth
1 pinch of sea salt

Halve romaine lettuce, boil semi-soft in water, drain, gather together and put in an oven-proof mould. Steam the onion slightly without fat and spread it on the lettuce. Add vegetable broth and sea salt and roast in the oven for 30–40 min.

Endive
1 large endive head

Prepare just like romaine lettuce.

Steamed chicory
2 heads chicory
½ teaspoon health-food store vegetable fat*
3 tablespoons vegetable broth
1 pinch of sea salt
marjoram, thyme
some butter* or olive oil* or nut spread*

Halve chicory and layer them in the pan. Add heated vegetable fat* and vegetable broth to the chicory, season and steam covered on low heat for ½ hour. If permitted, spread melted butter* or olive oil* or nut spread* on the prepared vegetables.

Chard (Swiss Chard) with Béchamel sauce
3 Swiss chards
½ dl vegetable broth
A little lemon juice or 1 tablespoon almond puree*
1 pinch of sea salt
tarragon, parsley and chives
Béchamel sauce* (see recipe on page 87)

Cut the Swiss chards into pieces of 3 cm, cook covered on low heat for ½ to ¾ hour until soft with the vegetable broth and lemon juice or almond puree*. Season and mix the fresh vegetables with Béchamel sauce*.

Stalk celery
3–4 stalks celery
½ onion, chopped
some apple, finely chopped
1 dl vegetable broth
1 teaspoon almond puree*
1 pinch of sea salt
optional Kelpamare
celery greens

Cut the celery into 8 cm long pieces and place in a pan. Slightly steam onion and apple without fat and spread on the celery. Add vegetable broth and almond puree* and cook soft for ½ to ¾ hour. Season.

Baked fennel with cream cheese sauce*
1 large or 2 small fennel
1 pinch of sea salt
pepper
some drops of lemon juice
1 cream cheese*

Quarter the fennel and steam it semi-soft in a little water. Pull apart the individual layers of the fennel and put them into an over-proof mould. Drip on lemon juice, salt and pepper. Stir the cream cheese* with 2 tablespoons of fennel stock and spread on the vegetables. Bake in a hot oven.

Vegetable curry
1 tablespoon sunflower oil*
1 spring onion
200 g vegetables (e.g. leeks, carrots, courgettes, asparagus)
½ teaspoon wholegrain flour*
1 knife tip (or more, as desired) curry powder
½ teaspoon vegetable broth
½ orange
1 teaspoon sultanas
1 pinch of whole sugar (Sucanat)
sea salt, pepper

Cut the spring onion into fine rings and cook in slightly heated oil. Sprinkle on flour and curry powder and add the vegetable broth. Add the cut small vegetables and steam covered for approx. 15 minutes. Reserve two or three wedges of the orange, squeeze the rest and place the sultanas in the juice. When the vegetables are soft, add the sultanas and orange juice, let the mixture become hot and season with sugar, salt and pepper. Serve and spread the orange wedges on top.

Steamed carrots
3–4 carrots
1 dl vegetable broth
1 teaspoon almond puree*
1 pinch of fruit sugar and sea salt each
marjoram, thyme, rosemary, parsley

Steam the carrots cut in slices or pegs in the vegetable broth for 30–45 min. Add the almond puree* if desired. Season and sprinkle on the chopped parsley.

Peas and carrots
(if tolerated and permitted)
100 g fresh garden peas, shelled
1 dl vegetable broth
marjoram, thyme, lovage, parsley, chives
150 g sliced carrots, prepared according to the recipe for steamed carrots

Cook peas in the vegetable broth until soft. Season. Mix carrots and peas or alternate them on the platter.

Peas, French style
(if tolerated and permitted)
¼ head of lettuce or romaine lettuce
150–200 g peas, shelled
1 dl vegetable broth
1 pinch of sea salt
parsley, chives marjoram, thyme, lovage
10 g nut spread*
1 teaspoon wholegrain flour*

Steam the lettuce or romaine lettuce cut into fine strips with the peas in the vegetable broth on very low heat until soft. Season. Mix nut spread* with wholegrain flour, add and boil briefly.

Steamed snow peas (sugar peas)/ mangetouts
200 g snow peas
1 dl vegetable broth
1 pinch of sea salt
1 pinch of fruit sugar
some parsley or lovage
chives, marjoram, thyme
fresh butter* or vegetable margarine* or nut spread*

Steam sugar peas and herbs covered in the vegetable broth for ½ to ¾ hour. Season. If permitted, add fresh butter* or health-food store vegetable fat*, olive oil* or nut spread* before serving.

Green beans
250 g beans
some garlic
savory, parsley
1–2 tomatoes
1 pinch of sea salt
some caraway, marjoram, lovage

Steam the beans, finely diced tomatoes and herbs for approx. 1 hour, add some water if necessary. Season.

Steamed celery root (celeriac)
½ celery root (celeriac)
1 dl vegetable broth
1 pinch of sea salt
some lemon juice, marjoram
1 teaspoon almond puree*
very fine slices of apple, nuts

Pour vegetable broth over the diced celery root (celeriac) and cook until soft, ½ to ¾ hour. Season. Enrich with almond puree* and steam with some apple slices if desired. Sprinkle with chopped nuts before serving.

Celery root (celeriac) with Béchamel sauce*
Prepare 1 small celery root (celeriac) as described above and finally mix with Béchamel sauce* (see recipe page 87).

Red beets
Cut off the root tips and leaves to approx. 2 cm and wash well without damaging the skin.
350 g red beets
1 dl vegetable broth
1 pinch of fruit sugar and 1 pinch of sea salt
¼ laurel leaf, lovage, caraway, nutmeg
a very little garlic, parsley, a little lemon juice, lemon balm
1 tablespoon wholegrain flour*, mixed cold
1 tablespoon almond puree

Cook the red beets soft in the pressure cooker for approx. 25 min. Peel and cut into thin slices. Mix well with the herbs and spices in the vegetable broth and cook slightly for 15 min. To bind, stir in the wholegrain flour* and finally add the almond puree*.

Jerusalem artichokes
250 g Jerusalem artichokes
some vegetable broth
1 pinch of sea salt
basil
1 teaspoon almond puree*

Cook the Jerusalem artichoke like potatoes in the peel (see recipe page 82). Peel, slice and steam until soft in the vegetable broth. Season and mix in the almond puree* to refine.
You can also prepare the Jerusalem artichoke with Béchamel sauce* (see recipe page 87) and some ground cheese*.

Stewed tomatoes
4–5 tomatoes
½ tablespoon olive oil*
½ onion
fruit sugar
1 pinch of sea salt
a little garlic, rosemary, marjoram, basil
1 tablespoon corn starch (optional)
parsley or chives or dill

Slightly brown onion and fruit sugar in olive oil in the skillet. Douse the tomatoes with boiling water and peel them, cut them into pieces, add them to the onions and steam the mixture until it has thickened a little. Add garlic and spices and finish cooking; for binding, add the corn starch. Sprinkle plenty of chopped parsley or other herbs on the prepared tomatoes.

Steamed tomatoes
2–3 tomatoes
1 pinch of sea salt
10 g health-food store vegetable fat*
¼ onion, chopped
herbes de Provence (basil, rosemary, thyme, sage), parsley

Steam onion lightly without fat. Put the halved tomatoes on a greased tray or overproof mould. Put small pieces of vegetable fat* on each tomato half, and spread the steamed onion and herbs on it. Steam briefly in the oven. As desired, some tomatoes may be pureed or very finely chopped, mixed with cream*, boiled quickly and spread on the prepared tomatoes.

Stuffed tomatoes
2–3 tomatoes
1 teaspoon rice per tomato
1 pinch of sea salt
butter* or health-food store vegetable fat* or olive oil* or nut spread*
some onion and garlic
rosemary, marjoram, thyme, basil
bay leaf, nutmeg
vegetable broth (optional)

Cut off the top of the tomatoes and hollow them out. Chop the tomato pulp and mix with 1 teaspoon uncooked rice and the herbs and spices. Fill in the mass, add butter flakes* or olive oil* or nut spread* and then put on the cut-off lids. Bake in the oven at moderate heat for 20–30 min.

Tomatoes à la Provençale
2 tomatoes
1 pinch of sea salt
1 tablespoon chopped parsley
1 tablespoon breadcrumbs

Halve tomatoes, sprinkle with sea salt, and place on a tray. Mix breadcrumbs and parsley and spread on the tomatoes with a spoon. Bake in the oven for 15 min.

Courgettes with tomatoes
½ onion, chopped
300 g courgettes
50 g tomatoes
1 pinch of sea salt
garlic, rosemary, marjoram, thyme, basil
parsley, chives, dill
some maize flour (optional)
1 teaspoon almond puree*

79

Steam the onion without fat. Dice the courgettes, peel the tomatoes and dice them as well. Add both vegetables to the onions and let them roast until soft. Season. If there is too much liquid, add some stirred-up maize flour and 1 teaspoon almond puree* before serving.

Peperoni, green, yellow or red
These are very well suitable as an addition to other dishes, but some liver patients find them indigestible.
150–200 g peperoni
½ tablespoon olive oil*
½ onion, chopped
1 pinch of sea salt
garlic, rosemary, marjoram, thyme, basil, parsley

Cut peperoni in strips and steam them together with onion, herbs and spices in olive oil in the covered pan for at least ½ hour.

Ratatouille
50 g peperoni
100 g courgettes
50 g aubergines
1 tomato
½ onion, chopped
some garlic
1 tablespoon olive oil*
1 pinch of sea salt
rosemary, marjoram, thyme, basil, parsley

Dice peperoni, courgettes, aubergines and tomato (peeled). Steam onion and garlic in olive oil, add vegetables and steam covered for 1 hour. Season. If there is too much juice, let it thicken while covered.

Artichokes
1 artichokes
¾ l water
1 tablespoon lemon juice
1 pinch of sea salt

Cut off the stalks close to the artichokes. Remove the bottom-most hard leaves and cut off the tips. Halve and cut out the heart; wash under running water and rub the cut surface with lemon juice. Boil water, add lemon juice and sea salt and cook the artichoke soft in it for approx. ¾ h. Drain it and prepare it on a warm platter with a serviette. Serve with yoghurt dressing (see recipe page 69).

Asparagus
½ bunch of asparagus
1 l water
1 pinch of sea salt
grated cheese*
nut spread*

Wash the asparagus and peel it completely. Green asparagus can be left almost whole. Boil water, cook the asparagus until soft (20–30 min.), take out with a perforated spoon and prepare on a platter with a serviette. Sprinkle with grated cheese* and pour liquid nut spread* over the dish.
As a variation, serve with remoulade sauce* (see recipe page 89).

Cauliflower or broccoli
1 small cauliflower or
250 g broccoli
1 teaspoon olive oil*
1 garlic clove
1 dl vegetable broth
sea salt, pepper

Cut off the leaves and stalk below the flower. Peel the stalk and cut into larger pieces; divide the flower into florets. Lightly brown the chopped garlic clove in olive oil*, add cauliflower or broccoli and steam along briefly. Douse with the vegetable broth and then cook for approx. 5 minutes. Season with salt and pepper. If permitted, briefly roast pine nuts or sliced almond without fat in a pan and spread on the vegetables.

Kohlrabi with herbs
1 kohlrabi
1 dl vegetable broth
1 tablespoon tender kohlrabi leaves, chopped
Béchamel sauce* (see recipe page 87)

Cut kohlrabi into 4 pieces, then into fine slices, and cook in the vegetable broth, covered, for ½–¾ hour. Add the kohlrabi leaves before serving.
Mix the Béchamel sauce* (see recipe page 87) with various chopped herbs and prepare on the cooked kohlrabi.

Corn on the cob
(chew very well, otherwise hard to digest)
1 corn cob
½ l salt water
1–2 tablespoons quark or vegetable margarine*

Use only corn cobs with tender and milky kernels. Remove the husks and strings. Cook the corn cob soft in salt water for 10–20 min. and serve it on a hot plate with vegetable margarine* or quark.

Salads of cooked vegetables

These dishes are only permitted for the stage-III and IV diets.

Carrots, celery, red beet, beans, cauliflower, broccoli, courgettes, beet greens or Swiss chard are particularly suitable for these salads.

The vegetables are cooked soft in vegetable broth or water, drained and cut small (dice, slices, florets, strips). Serve with salad dressing, yoghurt sauce* or mayonnaise*. Use onions and chopped herbs as spice.

Potato salad
200 g potatoes
½ dl vegetable broth
1 tablespoon mayonnaise
½ tablespoon chopped onions
borage, chives, parsley, lemon balm, marjoram, thyme, dill

Cook the potatoes until soft in the pressure cooker, peel while hot and slice. Pour the heated vegetable broth on them and let them stand for a little, then mix in the mayonnaise. Season with onions and herbs.

Potato salad with cucumbers
1 large potato
¼ cucumber
2 tablespoon yoghurt sauce
½ garlic clove
dill or borage, chives, parsley, onion

Prepare the potato as described above. Grate the peeled cucumber with a coarse grater and add to the potato. Mix with yoghurt sauce and season with onions and herbs.
Rub the salad bowl with the garlic clove before serving.

Salade niçoise
1 cooked potato
1 small tomato
radishes
some slices of cucumber
1 tablespoon oil
½ tablespoon lemon juice
1 pinch of sea salt
parsley, chives or dill, lemon balm, borage
some leaves of head lettuce

Slice the potato, tomato and radish and dress with a salad dressing of oil*, lemon juice, sea salt and herbs. Right before serving, mix the lettuce leaves with the salad or prepare the salad on the head-lettuce leaves.

Rice salad
50 g rice
2 dl water
2 tablespoon quark sauce
½ tablespoon chopped onions
¼ tomato
chives, parsley or basil
some salad leaves

Cook the rice in water, rinse it briefly and let it cool off. Add the onion, finely diced tomato and herbs to the quark sauce. Mix the rice with the sauce and prepare on salad leaves.

Celery root (celeriac) salad with soy mayonnaise*
½ small celery root (celeriac)
½–1 tablespoon lemon juice
2 walnuts
¼ apple (optional)
1 pinch of sea salt
1 tablespoon soy mayonnaise* (see recipe page 70)

Cut the raw celery root (celeriac) into match-thin strips or grate it. Drip on lemon juice to prevent browning. Add the coarsely chopped walnuts and the grated apple and mix with the mayonnaise*.

Vegetable brawn
2½ dl vegetable broth
2 g agar-agar
some drops of lemon juice
some Kelpamare
fresh slices of cucumber
cubes of tomato
cooked broccoli florets
cooked peas
cooked, finely chopped beans
1 pinch of sea salt

Agar-agar is plant-based gelatine powder that is used for vegetable and fruit aspics, sauces and puddings, etc. instead of animal gelatine.

Add agar-agar powder to the lukewarm vegetable broth and heat slowly until the gelling agent is well dissolved. Season with sea salt, lemon juice and Kelpamare. Pour a little brawn into the rinsed moulds and let it harden. Garnish with vegetable slices, add brawn again, let it harden, and so forth until the moulds are filled.

Turn over the cooled brawns and serve on salad leaves.

Potato dishes

Potatoes in their skins
2–4 small potatoes
water
1 pinch of sea salt

Brush and wash potatoes. Fill pan with steamer insert or wire screen with water to the insert, add potatoes, cover and cook for 30 to 40 minutes. They will be soft within 8–10 minutes in the pressure cooker.

Baked potatoes/jacket potatoes
3–4 small potatoes
1 tablespoon oil*
nut spread*

Brush and wash the potatoes. On the top, score the peel 3–4 times, brush with oil* and bake them on a greased sheet at medium heat for 30–40 min. Put a dab of nut spread* on each of the finished potatoes. For liver patients, oil should not be heated when baking and be absorbed by the potatoes. So, do not brush on.

Quark potatoes
3–4 small potatoes
50 g lean quark
1–2 tablespoons milk or cream*
chives or caraway or marjoram
1 pinch of sea salt

Cut a groove into the top of the potatoes and prepare them as for baked potatoes (leave out the oil). For the stuffing, stir quark with milk or cream* until foamy and add spices.
Use a spoon to spread it on the groove of the baked potatoes or apply with a cream bag.

Caraway potatoes
2–3 medium-sized, longish, narrow potatoes
1 teaspoon caraway
1 pinch of sea salt
1 tablespoon olive oil*

Brush off the potatoes, wash them and cut them in half on the short axis. Mix caraway with sea salt and sprinkle on the cuts. Put the potatoes on a greased tray with the cut down, brush with oil* (see for baked potatoes) and bake at medium heat for ¾ hour.

Bouillon potatoes
250 g potatoes
1–2 dl vegetable broth
1 pinch of sea salt
lovage, thyme
10 g butter*, health-food store vegetable fat*, olive oil* or nut spread*

Wash potatoes, peel, halve or cut into pieces and cook until soft in the vegetable broth with sea salt and the spices. Spread butter*, olive oil* or nut spread* on the prepared potatoes.

Cream potatoes*
200 g potatoes
onion, chopped
1 dl vegetable broth
1 pinch of sea salt
½ dl cream* or milk
thyme, nutmeg, miso
parsley

Peel potatoes, slice, steam them briefly with the onion without fat and cook until soft with the vegetable broth and spices. Add cream* or milk. Sprinkle the prepared potatoes with chopped parsley.

Potatoes with tomatoes
200 g potatoes
½ kl. onion
1 dl vegetable broth
1 kl. tomatoes
1 pinch of sea salt
1 tablespoon sesame cream*
Marjoram, rosemary or thyme

Let the chopped onion and peeled, sliced potatoes steam briefly without fat, then cook them semi-soft with the vegetable broth. Cut the peeled tomato into wedges, add and finish cooking. Season. Add the cream* before serving.

Potato puree
4 potatoes
water
dried tomatoes
butter*, health-food store vegetable fat*, olive oil* or nut spread*

Wash the potatoes, peel, cut into pieces and steam them soft with a little water. Press onto a warm platter directly through a potato ricer. Add melted butter*, olive oil* or nut spread* and garnish with finely cut dried tomatoes.

Mashed Potatoes
4 potatoes
water
1 dl milk
nutmeg
1 tablespoon cream* (optional)
1 pinch of sea salt
finely chopped marjoram, finely chopped caraway, nutmeg
garlic
dried tomatoes

Peel potatoes, cut them into pieces and cook them soft in the steam. Strain through the potato ricer. Heat milk, add the potato mash, stir until foamy and season. If desired, enrich with cream*. Serve on a hot platter, garnished with finely cut dried tomatoes.

Roast potatoes*
2 small potatoes
water
1 pinch of sea salt
1 dl vegetable broth
1–2 tablespoons sesame cream* or nut spread*
nutmeg, thyme
parsley

Peel and halve potatoes and cook them semi-soft in the steam. Put them on an oven-proof platter with the cut side down. Pour on vegetable broth, season and roast in the oven until the liquid has thickened. Add cream* or nut spread* and continue roasting until the potatoes are lightly browned. Serve with the cut facing up and sprinkle with chopped parsley.

Potato slices with spinach
1 large potato
1 dl vegetable broth
1 pinch of sea salt
100 g spinach
butter*, olive oil* or nut spread*
garlic, parsley, chives
optional peppermint or sage, nutmeg

Cut the peeled potato lengthwise into 1 cm- thick slices and cook carefully until soft. Place on a buttered tray. Prepare the spinach like leaf spinach (see recipe page 76), season and distribute among the potatoes. Sprinkle with grated cheese* if desired and brush with olive oil* or apply dabs of butter* or nut spread*. Briefly bake in the oven.

Potato "Goulash"
1 onion
1 large potato
1 green peperoni
1–2 dl water
1 pinch of sea salt
marjoram, thyme, nutmeg

Finely dice the onion and potato, cut the peperoni into pieces and cover with water in a pan. Cook until soft, approx. 15 minutes. Season well and serve.

Ayurveda potatoes
(a pretty, very aromatic dish that yields 3–4 helpings)
5 large potatoes
½ soy drink
1 package of soy crème (substitute for crème fraîche)
1 bunch each of fresh dill, fresh chives and fresh parsley
juice of ½ lemon
1–2 teaspoons turmeric
½ teaspoon curry
1 pinch of sea salt
soy sauce

Cut the well-brushed potatoes into thick slices and cook them for approx. 5 minutes. In the meantime, slowly heat the soy drink in a pan, mixed with the soy crème (do not boil!). Stir in turmeric, curry and sea salt to taste and season with soy sauce. Put the potato slices in the sauce and simmer for approx. 10 minutes. Finally, sprinkle the fresh, finely chopped herbs on the potatoes and serve at once.

Cereal Dishes

Japanese rice
80 g wholegrain rice
1½–2 dl vegetable bouillon
1 pinch of sea salt
10 g butter*, health-food store vegetable fat*, olive oil* or nut spread*
1 small peeled onion, stuck with a bay leaf and a clove

Put the rice in the cooking bouillon with the onion and boil for 40 minutes. Let it cool off. Heat the rice again in the oven and top with melted butter*, vegetable margarine* or nut spread* before serving.

Risotto
80 g wholegrain rice

1 tablespoon chopped onion
2 dl vegetable broth or water
1 pinch of sea salt
dried mushrooms
fresh herbs as desired, rosemary
10 g fresh butter*, health-food store vegetable fat*, olive oil* or nut spread*
10 g Parmesan cheese* (optional)

Steam the rice with the onion until the rice is translucent. Add the vegetable broth or water hot and cook al dente (30–40 minutes). Add the finely chopped, dried mushrooms and herbs and cook together a little. Before serving, mix in butter*, olive oil*, health-food store vegetable fat* or nut spread* and grated parmesan* with a fork.

Saffron rice
Prepare like risotto. Dissolve a knife tip of saffron powder in a little bouillon and add.

Riz creole with vegetables
80 g wholegrain rice
1 tablespoon vegetables (leeks, celery, carrots), finely chopped in cubes
2 dl vegetable broth
1 pinch of sea salt
bay leaf, cloves, optional nutmeg
freshly chopped herbs as desired

Briefly steam rice and vegetables, add hot vegetable broth and spices and cook for 30–45 min.

Tomato rice
80 g wholegrain rice
1 tablespoon chopped onion
garlic, pressed
1 large tomato
approx. 1 dl vegetable broth
1 pinch of sea salt
rosemary, marjoram, nutmeg, optional basil
sugar (Sucanat)
10 g butter* or olive oil*

Steam onion, garlic and rice until the rice is translucent. Add peeled, diced tomato. Add vegetable broth and spices and cook for 30–45 min. Before serving, mix in fresh butter* or olive oil*.

Rice with courgettes
80 g wholegrain rice
1 tablespoon chopped onion
150 g tender courgettes
1 pinch of sea salt
1½ dl vegetable broth or water
soy sauce, freshly chopped dill
10 g butter*, olive oil* or nut spread*

Dice courgettes. Prepare dish as for tomato rice.

Rice with spinach
80 g wholegrain rice
100 g spinach
onion, chopped
2 dl vegetable broth or water
1 pinch of sea salt
nutmeg and peppermint
10 g fresh butter* or olive oil* or nut spread*

Coarsely cut spinach. Prepare dish as for tomato rice

Rice with peas (Risi bisi)
80 g wholegrain rice
150 g garden peas, shelled
onion, chopped
1 pinch each of fruit sugar and sea salt
½ dl vegetable broth
1½–2 dl water
10 g butter*, olive oil* or nut spread*
parsley

Steam onion with fruit sugar and sea salt. Add the peas and steam briefly, then add vegetable broth and cook the peas until soft. Prepare risotto (according to the above recipe) in a separate pan. Mix in the cooked peas. Before serving, top with butter*, olive oil* or nut spread* and chopped parsley.

Rice gratin with tomatoes
80 g wholegrain rice
2 small tomatoes
onion, chopped
2 tablespoons vegetables (leek, celery, carrots)
1½ dl vegetable broth
1 pinch of sea salt
parsley, lovage
5 g butter* or olive oil*

Briefly steam onion and very finely diced vegetables, add the rice and continue cooking until it is translucent. Douse in hot vegetable broth, season and cook for 30–45 min. Put the finished rice and the sliced tomatoes into an oven-proof mould in layers, top with dabs of butter* or brush on olive oil* and bake in the oven for 10 min.

Indian rice
80 g wholegrain rice
2 dl vegetable broth
1 pinch of sea salt
1 small banana
1 small apple
1 tablespoon raisins
1 teaspoon sunflower seeds
1 teaspoon sesame seeds
saffron, curry, fresh ginger root

Cook rice with vegetable broth and 1 pinch of sea salt until not quite soft (approx. 30–40 minutes). Mix the sliced banana, the peeled and sliced apple and the raisins into the rice and continue boiling for 5–10 min. Season with saffron, curry and ginger root to taste. Sprinkle with sunflower seeds and lightly dry-roasted sesame seeds.

Semolina
50 g semolina
3 dl milk
2 dl water
1 pinch of sea salt
1 tablespoon sesame cream
1 tablespoon each of fruit sugar and cinnamon

Stir semolina into the boiling liquid, add salt and cook for 15–20 min. Sprinkle the cream and fruit sugar mixed with cinnamon onto the prepared semolina mash.

Polenta
50 g maize semolina, medium-fine
3 dl water
nutmeg
1 pinch of sea salt
½ tablespoon fresh butter*, olive oil* or nut spread*

Boil water and stir in the maize. Boil for 5 min. on low heat, stirring constantly. Season and continue boiling for 45–60 min. on low heat. For the stage-IV diet, add butter*, olive oil* or nut spread* before serving. As desired, you may also add onion slices roasted without fat.

Millet risotto
50 g millet
1 tablespoon chopped onion
1½ dl vegetable broth
½ onion
1 pinch of sea salt

Steam onion and hot-rinsed millet until glazed, add the hot vegetable broth and salt and cook for 20 min. Before serving, top with onion strips roasted without fat.

Millet risotto with vegetables
40 g millet
1 tablespoon chopped onion
2 tablespoons finely chopped vegetable cubes (leek, celery, carrots or carrots and peas)
1½ dl vegetable broth
1 pinch of sea salt
Miso
rosemary
10 g fresh butter* or nut spread*

Steam onion, vegetable dice and hot-rinsed millet until glazed. Add hot vegetable broth, season and boil for 20 min. Before serving, top with dabs of butter or nut spread* if desired.

Coarse-ground grain mash
2 tablespoons coarse-ground grain (wheat, oats, rye)
3 tablespoons water
1 pinch of sea salt

Soak the coarse-ground grain for 12 hours. Then boil in the water for 10 min. or cook for ½ hour in a bain-marie.

Pasta, spaghetti, macaroni, etc.
Liver patients should not use egg pasta. Today, there also are outstanding wholegrain pasta, soy pasta and spelt pasta in addition to the well-known Italian pasta products made from wheat. Additionally, there are any number of sauces, which usually contain much too much fat for liver patients (oil, butter, cheese, cream).
The best-tolerated pasta products are cooked *al dente* with a classic or simple tomato sauce (see recipes in the chapter on "Sauces").

Spätzle or Knöpfli (without egg)
60 g wholegrain flour
20 g soy flour
1 dl water
1 l water
1 tablespoon sea salt
1 tablespoon health-food store vegetable fat or olive oil*
strips of onion
chives and parsley

Mix wholegrain and soy flour well with water and tap it until the dough forms bubbles. Then let it rest for at least 1 hour. Boil water with sea salt. Rub the dough in portions through a coarse screen into the boiling water or put it onto a small cutting board and cut fine strips with a knife and drop them into the boiling water.
Let the Knöpfli or Spätzle simmer until they come to the surface. Take them out with a skimmer and prepare them on a hot platter. As desired, garnish with onion strips roasted in olive oil* (or entirely without fat), chives and parsley.

Sauces

Sauces are a difficult section for liver patients, since almost all sauce recipes contain a lot of fat (butter, oil, cream), cheese and eggs. We have put together a few permitted sauces here, with some recipes deviating from the classical ones – but still tasting outstandingly!

Béchamel sauce
For 4 persons:
2 tablespoons wheat flour
½ l soy milk
1 bay leaf
1 finely grated onion
2 teaspoons red miso
1 pinch each of pepper and paprika
chopped parsley

Briefly brown the flour without fat until it gives off a toasted flavour. Let it cool a

little, then add the soy milk while stirring constantly. Add the bay leaf and onion and let everything boil for about 5 min. Stir in the miso, remove the bay leaf and season the sauce with pepper and paprika. Sprinkle with chopped parsley.
(Miso is a fermented soy bean paste that is great for seasoning and tastes like the popular soy sauce. Be careful to buy non-GMO soy products.)

Béchamel sauce 2*
This version is a little less "exotic" and closer to the well-known old recipe. It must, however, be used only if milk is permitted.

For 4 persons:
2–3 tablespoons wheat flour
1 l milk*
1 bay leaf
1 tablespoon vegetable broth
1 grated onion
1 pinch each of sea salt, nutmeg and freshly ground white pepper
chopped parsley

Briefly roast the flour without fat until it is aromatic (it must not turn dark), then let it cool slightly. Add the milk, bay leaf, vegetable broth and onion while stirring constantly and boil the mixture. Season. After approx. 5 minutes, remove the bay leaf and serve the sauce sprinkled with parsley. This basic sauce can be used to make many versions, e.g.

Horseradish sauce: at the end, add 10 g finely grated horseradish and cook the sauce for another 5 min.

Caper sauce: Season the finished sauce with whole or chopped capers and lemon juice.

Olive sauce: Briefly cook the sauce with 4–5 teaspoons tomato pulp and 2 teaspoons chopped olives. If required, season with a knife point of cayenne pepper.

Herb sauce: Mix plenty of finely chopped herbs such as parsley, lovage, chervil, basil, estragon, oregano, etc. into the finished sauce.

Champignon sauce: Mix 3–4 teaspoons of very finely chopped raw champignons into the finished sauce and season with lemon juice.

Tomato sauce, classic recipe
½ tablespoon health-food store vegetable fat*
1 tablespoon onion
½ garlic clove, pressed
2 tablespoons carrot, celery, leek

2 small tomatoes
1 pinch of sea salt
1 pinch of fruit or whole sugar
1 teaspoon tomato puree
1½ dl vegetable broth or water
rosemary, thyme

Steam chopped onion, pressed garlic and coarsely cut vegetables well in the health-food store vegetable fat* (steam without fat for the stage-III diet). Steam the tomatoes cut into pieces and the tomato puree as well. Add vegetable broth or water, season and simmer for ½ hour. Strain if desired.

Tomato sauce, simple
3 tomatoes
1 pinch each of sea salt and whole sugar (Sucanat)
chives, basil
1 tablespoon olive oil*

Cut tomatoes into pieces, steam gently, season and strain as desired. For the stage-IV diet, add some olive oil before serving.

Mayonnaise without animal protein*
See recipe on page 70

Remoulade sauce*
For 4 persons:

Make mayonnaise without animal protein (see page 70) and mix with 1 tablespoon chopped cornichons, some capers and chopped parsley. Garnish with tomato dice.

Sandwiches

Sandwiches are generally popular as appetizers or for a summer dinner, and to take along on hikes and trips or as lunch at the office.

Spreads and ingredients can be used in any number of new ways, and different wholegrain bread types are available as well, some already pre-cut.

The recipes here are calculated for 4 persons.

Basic spreads
In the strict diet, only spread some quark on the bread rolls and fill with raw food.

Guacamole (avocado mousse)
2 ripe avocados
juice of ½ lemon
½ small chopped onion
2 garlic cloves, pressed
sea salt and white pepper

Mash the removed pulp of the avocados with the lemon juice in a blender. Mix in onion and garlic and season with sea salt and white pepper. If desired, stir in 1 tablespoon soy cream.

Sweet avocado mousse
1 ripe avocado
4 tablespoons freshly pressed orange juice
1 tablespoon honey
1 knife tip ginger powder

Mash the removed pulp of the avocado by squeezing or blending and mix in the other ingredients. Serve at once.

Tofu spread with nuts
250 g tofu, pureed
2 finely chopped spring onions
50 g nuts (hazelnuts, walnuts, almonds, cashews)
sea salt and white pepper

Lightly roast the nuts in the oven or a dry pan, let them cool off and grind them. Mix with the pureed tofu and onions. Season with sea salt and pepper.

Quark spread with herbs*
100 g quark
10 g butter*, health-food store vegetable fat* or nut spread*
miso
caraway, chives or herbs such as dill, borage, lovage, basil, oregano, peppermint etc.

Stir quark and health-food store vegetable fat* until of a creamy consistency, season and add individual herbs or a mix for variety.

Garnishes
Bread with spread can be garnished in the following ways:
with raw carrots or celery, tomatoes, fresh cucumbers, radish, cress, onion rings, nuts, parsley, chives etc.

89

Desserts

These recipes are all intended for 4 persons.

Desserts should be eaten with great restraint; they are not permitted for the stage-I and -II diets. Instead, use honey (acacia honey is particularly good), peach honey, maple syrup, agave juice or whole sugar (Sucanat, Panela, etc.), which is not suitable for all sweet dishes because of its own strong taste. Do not eat any sweet dishes with lots of sugar, eggs and cream. There are many tasty alternatives, however!

Fruit salad
2 tablespoons honey
1 dl water
1–2 dl grape juice or fruit juice
1–2 tablespoons lemon juice
600 g apricots or peaches
melons
apples
pears (soft type)
red cherries, pitted
all sorts of berries

Heat water with honey, grape juice and lemon juice and let the mixture cool. Thinly slice fruits, depending on season, and add them to the syrup.

Filled melons
2 small melons
fruit salad as per recipe above

Halve the melons, hollow them out and fill them with the fruit salad.

Fruit jelly
3 dl water or grape juice
2 tablespoons honey
10 g agar-agar, powdered
7 dl juice of oranges or berries.

Agar-agar is a plant-based gelatine powder that is used for vegetable and fruit spreads, sauces and puddings, etc. instead of animal gelatine.

Mix water well with honey and agar-agar and heat on low heat while stirring constantly until the agar-agar has completely dissolved. Mix fruit juice into it and serve immediately in glasses or dessert cups. Season as desired and garnish with sesame cream* (see recipe, page 71).

Applesauce
800 g apples
2 dl water or fruit juice
2 tablespoons honey
cinnamon or lemon peel
1 dl sesame cream*

Remove stem and calyx from the apples, cut the apples into pieces, cook them with the water or fruit juice and honey until soft and strain them. Mix with cinnamon or lemon peel zest (from untreated lemons only!). To enrich, serve sesame-cream with the apple mash.

Apple or pear compote
800 g apples or pears
2–3 dl water or fruit juice
1 tablespoon honey
lemon zest (from untreated lemons) or a little cinnamon

Peel apples or pears, remove the cores and cut them into wedges. Bring water or juice to a boil, add honey and lemon peel or cinnamon and cook the apples or pears in it until soft.

Stuffed apples, steamed
800 g apples
½ l water or fruit juice
1 tablespoon honey
¼ cinnamon stalks
quince, raspberry or currant jelly or raisins and grapes with a little honey

Boil water or fruit juice with honey and cinnamon stalks. Peel apples, halve them, hollow them out, put them into the hot juice in portions and cook them. Cook slowly until soft. Lift out with the skimmer and place on a flat platter with the cut surface up. Fill the apples with the desired jelly or the raisin-grape-honey mix.

Stuffed apples* in the oven
4 large or 8 small apples
4 tablespoons ground hazelnuts
2 tablespoons currants
4 tablespoon sesame cream*
2 tablespoon honey
lemon zest (from untreated lemon)
10 g butter*, vegetable margarine* or nut spread*
1 tablespoon wholegrain flour
1–2 dl fruit juice

Mix hazelnuts, currants, cream, honey and lemon peel, fill them into the prepared apples (core removed, peel scored) and put the apples into a casserole. Spread butter*, vegetable margarine* or nut spread* and sugar on the apples and pour fruit juice over them to 1 cm. Bake in the oven for 20–30 min.

Dried fruit salad with grapes and pine nuts
200 g dried figs
200 g dates
200 g dried apples
400 g white grapes
juice of 1 lemon
2 tablespoons honey
50 g pine nuts

Chop the dried fruit, halve half of the grapes and squeeze the others. Put all fruits in a dish. Mix the juice of the lemon and the grapes with the honey well and pour it over the fruits. Cool before serving. Roast the pine nuts dry and spread them on the fruit salad.

Strawberry or raspberry cream*
300 g berries
vanilla cream
1–2 dl sesame cream*

Prepare a vanilla cream according to the recipe on page 92 and mix with the mixed or pureed berries. Fold in sesame cream* or serve separately.

Lemon cream*
¾ l milk*
1–2 lemons, untreated
1 tablespoon cornflour or arrowroot flour
3 tablespoons milk*
2 tablespoons honey
sesame cream* as desired

Boil the thinly peeled lemon peel with the milk, add the corn starch or arrowroot flour stirred with a little cold milk and the honey and boil again. Strain the cooled crème and add a few spoons of lemon juice, as well as sesame cream* as desired.

Orange crème*
prepare as lemon cream (see recipe above)

Orange brawn
5 dl orange juice
5 g agar-agar, powdered (vegetable gelatine)
1 tablespoon fruit sugar

Mix 3 dl orange juice, agar-agar and sugar well and heat on low heat while stirring continuously (do not boil), until the agar-agar has dissolved completely. Add the remaining orange juice and pour into cold-rinsed moulds. Cool.

Sesame bars
100 g Syramena sugar
2 tablespoons honey
100 g sesame seeds, not ground

Syramena sugar is a light whole-cane crystal sugar available in organic food stores. Heat the sugar in a dry pan and stir until a light caramel results. Add the liquid honey and mix well. Add the sesame and mix well again. Pour the mass into a mould or onto an oiled board, let it cool slightly and cut into squares or diamonds. Let cool.

Vanilla crème
1 vanilla pod
¼ l water
40 g wheat flour
3 tablespoon honey
approx. 200 ml soy milk

Cut open the vanilla pod with a pointed knife, scratch out the pulp and let everything boil up with the water. Put the wheat flour into the vanilla water while stirring constantly and let it swell into a thick mash. Let it cool a little, then stir in the honey and soy milk well. Depending on the amount of soy milk, you will get vanilla crème or vanilla sauce. Keep cool until serving.

Vanilla sauce
See vanilla crème (recipe above)

Almond-milk sauce
4 dl milk
50 g almonds or almond spread
2 tablespoons honey
1 tablespoon cornflour or arrowroot flour
2 tablespoons water

Boil milk with the peeled, ground almonds (or the almond spread) and honey. Stir cornflour or arrowroot flour in cold water and stir into the boiling milk. Mix the finished sauce well.

Rosehip sauce
70 g rosehip puree or rosehip pulp
2 dl water or grape juice
2 tablespoons honey
some drops of lemon juice (optional)

Boil the ingredients together, then add the lemon juice.

Red wine sauce
2 dl water
lemon or orange peel (from untreated fruits)
1 cinnamon stalk
1 clove
2 tablespoons honey
2 dl red grape juice
20 g almonds

Boil water, peel, spices and honey together for a few min., then strain. Add grape juice and heat (do not boil). Add peeled and sliced almonds.

Red fruit jelly
7 dl currant, raspberry or strawberry juice
3 dl red grape juice or water
70 g semolina
1 tablespoon cornflour

Boil berry juice and grape juice together, stir in semolina and cornflour and boil for 10 min. Fill into rinsed pudding mould and cool.
Serve with vanilla sauce (recipe page 92) or almond-milk sauce (recipe page 92).

Red fruit jelly, Danish style
1 kg berries (raspberries, currants, strawberries or pitted cherries, or all mixed)
1 l fruit juice (e.g. elderberry)
2 packs of agar-agar
honey as desired
½ teaspoon natural vanilla
sesame-cream* liquid

Put cleaned and possibly crushed fruits into a dish. Heat fruit juice with agar-agar as specified. Mix the fruits with honey and vanilla and pour the agar-agar liquid over them. Let the fruit jelly harden. Serve with liquid sesame cream*.

List of recipes

Almond milk	71		Celery root (celeriac) with	
Almond milk from			Béchamel sauce	78
fresh almonds	71		Cereal grains, sprouted	67
Almond-milk sauce	92		Chamomile tea	65
Almond-puree dressing	70		Champignon sauce	88
Alpine lady's-mantle tea	66		Chard (Swiss Chard) with	
Apple or pear compote	90		Béchamel sauce	77
Applesauce	90		Chervil soup	75
Apples, stuffed, in the oven	91		Chicory, steamed	77
Apples, stuffed, steamed	90		Coarse-ground grain mash	87
Artichokes	80		Corn on the cob	81
Asparagus	80		Courgettes with tomatoes	79
Avocado mousse (guacamole)	89		Cream dressing	69
Avocado mousse, sweet	89		Cream potatoes	83
Ayurveda potatoes	84			
			Endive	76
Bearberry leaf tea	66			
Béchamel sauce	87		Fennel, baked	
Béchamel sauce 2	88		with cream cheese sauce	77
Birchermuesli with			Flatulence tea	65
almond or sesame puree	66		Flax seed tea	65
Birchermuesli with			Fruit jelly	90
berries or stone fruit	67		Fruit juices	64
Birchermuesli with			Fruit salad	90
condensed milk	67		Fruit salad, dried, with grapes	
Birchermuesli with dried fruits	67		and pine nuts	91
Birchermuesli with orange juice	67			
Birchermuesli with various fruits	67		Garlic dressing	70
Birchermuesli with			Green beans	78
yoghurt or sour or buttermilk	66		Gruel to Go with Juices	65
Bitter tea	65		Guacamole (avocado mousse)	89
Bouillon potatoes	83			
Broccoli	80		Herbal soup	74
			Herb sauce	88
Caper sauce	88		Horseradish sauce	88
Caraway potatoes	83			
Carrots, steamed	77		Jacket potatoes/potatoes, baked	82
Cauliflower	80		Jerusalem artichokes	79
Celery root (celeriac) salad				
with soy mayonnaise	82		Knöpfli or Spätzle (without egg)	87
Celery root (celeriac), steamed	78		Kohlrabi with herbs	81

Lady's-mantle tea	66	Quark potatoes	82
Lavender tea	66	Quark sauce	69
Lemon-balm tea	65	Quark spread with herbs	89
Lemon cream	91		
Lemon dressing	69	Raspberry or strawberry crème	91
Lemon-peel tea	65	Ratatouille	80
Lettuce	76	Red beets	78
		Red fruit jelly	92
Mayonnaise without animal protein	88	Red fruit jelly, Danish style	92
		Red wine sauce	92
Mayonnaise with wholegrain soy flour instead of egg	70	Remoulade sauce	89
		Rice gratin with tomatoes	86
Melons, filled	90	Rice, Indian	86
Millet risotto	86	Rice, Japanese	85
Millet risotto with vegetables	87	Rice salad	82
Minestrone	76	Rice soup, clear	73
		Rice soup, thickened	73
Nut dressing	70	Rice with courgettes	85
		Rice with peas (Risi bisi)	86
Oat cream soup	74	Rice with spinach	85
Oat groats soup	74	Risi bisi (Rice with peas)	86
Oil dressing	69	Risotto	85
Olive sauce	88	Riz creole with vegetables	85
Orange-blossom tea	65	Roast potatoes	84
Orange brawn	91	Romaine lettuce	76
Orange crème	91	Rosehip sauce	92
Orange dressing	70	Rosehip tea	66
Pasta products	87	Saffron rice	85
Pear or apple compote	90	Salade niçoise	81
Peas and carrots	78	Sandwiches	89
Peas, French style	78	Sauerkraut salad	71
Peperoni, green, yellow or red	80	Semolina	86
Peppermint dressing	70	Semolina soup	74
Peppermint tea	65	Sesame bars	91
Pine nut milk	71	Sesame cream	71
Polenta	86	Sesame frappé/milkshake	72
Potatoes, Ayurveda style	84	Sesame milk	71
Potatoes, baked/jacket potatoes	82	Sesame-puree dressing	70
Potatoes in thier skins	82	Solidago tea	66
Potatoes, mashed	83	Soy milk	72
Potatoes with tomatoes	83	Spätzle or Knöpfli (without egg)	87
Potato "Goulash"	84		
Potato puree	83	Spinach, chopped	76
Potato salad	81	Spinach, whole leaves (and stems)	76
Potato salad with cucumbers	81		
Potato slices with spinach	84	Sprouted cereal grains	67
Potato soup	75	Stalk celery	77

Strawberry or raspberry cream	91	Vanilla crème	92
Sugar peas (snow peas)/ mangetouts, steamed	78	Vanilla sauce	92
		Various vegetable soups (carrots, spinach, broccoli)	75
Tofu spread with nuts	89	Vegetable bouillon	73
Tomatoes à la Provençale	79	Vegetable brawn	82
Tomatoes, steamed	79	Vegetable broth	73
Tomatoes, stewed	79	Vegetable curry	77
Tomatoes, stuffed	79	Vegetable Juices	64
Tomatoes with courgettes	79	Vervain tea	65
Tomato rice	85		
Tomato sauce, classic	88	Wormwood tea	65
Tomato sauce, simple	88		
Tomato soup	74	Yoghurt dressing	69
Tomato soup, summery	75		

Bibliography

Astrup, A. et al., "Dietary fibre added to very low calorie reduces hunger and alleviates constipation", *J-Obes*, Feb. 1990, vol 14 (2), pp. 109–12, ISSN: 0307–6565.

Attili, A. F. et al., "Dierand gallstones in Italy: the cross-sectional MICOL results", *Hepatology*, June 1998, vol. 27 (6), pp. 1492–8, ISSN: 0270–9139.

Bachmann, Robert M. et al., *Die Wassertherapie (praktische Anwendungen)*, Verlagsgesellschaft W. P. Sachon KG, Bad Wörishofen, ISBN: 3–923493.

Bae, C. Y. et al., "Clinical trial of American Heart Associatian step one diet for treatment of hypercholesterolemics", *J-Fam-Pract*, Sept. 1991, vol. 33 (3), pp. 249–54, ISSN: 0094–3509.

Barlow, C. W. et al., "Effects of therapy with diet and simvastatin on atherosclerosis in hypercholesterolemic patients", *Cardiovasc-Drugs-Ther.*, Oct. 1990, vol. 4 (5), pp. 1389–94, ISSN: 0920–3206.

Bell, L. P. et al., "Cholesterol-lowering effects of soluble-fibre cereals as part of a prudent diet for patients with mild to moderate hypercholesterolemia", *Am-J-Clin-Nutr.*, Dec. 1990, vol. 52 (6), pp. 1020–6, ISSN: 002–9165.

Bircher-Benner, M. O., "Vegetabile Heilkost. Wissenschaftliche Grundlagen für die Bewertung und die qualitative Zusammensetzung der vegetabilen Heilkost. Klin. Fortbildung", *Neue deutsche Klinik*, supplement, Verlag Urban & Schwarzenberg, Berlin and Vienna, 1933.

Bircher-Benner, M., "Vegetabile Heilkost. Klinische Fortbildungin", *Neue deutsche Klinik*, supplement, pp. 110–168, 1937.

Bircher-Benner, M. O., *Vom Werden des neuen Arztes*, Verlag Wilhelm Heine, Dresden 1938, new edition: *Mein Testament*, Bircher-Benner Verlag GmbH, Friedrichsdorf, 1984.

Bohn, H. and H. Runge, "Die Behandlung der Leberzirrhose mit Rohkost", *Zentralbl. f. Inn. Med.*, Verlag Johann Ambrosius Bartz, Leipzig, vol. 59, no. 11, pp. 193–199, 1938.

Bruch, S. W. et al., "The management of non- pigmented gallstones in children", *J-Pedia-Surg*, May 2000, vol. 35 (5), pp. 729–32, ISSN: 0022–3468.

Cabré, E. et al., "Short and long-term outcome of severe alcohol induced hepatitis treated with steroid or enteral nutrition: a multicenter randomised trial", *Hepatology*, July 2000, vol. 32 (1), pp. 36–42, ISSN: 0270–9139.

Campillo, B. et al., "Influence of liver failure, ascites, and energy expenditure on the response of oral nutrition in alcoholic liver cirrhosis", *Nutrition*, July–Aug 1997, vol. 13 (7–8), pp. 613–21, ISSN: 0899–9007.

Cara, L. et al., "Plasma lipid lowering effects of wheat germ in hypercholesterolemic subjects", *Plant-Foods-HumNutr*, Apr. 1991, vol. 41 (2), pp. 135–50, ISSN: 0921–9668.

Caroli Bosc, F. X. et al., "Cholelithiasis and dietary risk factors: an epidemiologic investigation in Vidauban, Southeast France", *Dig-Dis-Sci*, Sept. 1998, vol. 43 (9), pp. 2131–7, ISSN: 0163–2116.

Chang, Claude J. et al., "Mortality pattern of German vegetarians after 11 years of follow-up" (see comments), *Epidemiology*, Sept. 1992, vol. 3 (5), pp. 395–401, ISSN: 1044–3983.

Chang, Claude J. et al., "Dietary and life-style determinants of mortality among German vegetarians. Division of Epidemiology, German Cancer Research Center, Heidelberg", *Int-J-Epidemiol*, Apr. 1993, vol. 22 (2), pp. 228–36, ISSN: 0300–5771.

Christl, S. U. et al., "Fatty liver in adult celiac disease", *Deutsche Medizinische* Wochenschrift, 4 June 1999, vol. 124 (22), pp. 691–4, ISSN: 0012–0472.

Corrao, G. et al., "Exploring the role of diet in modifying the effect of known disease determinants: application to risk factors of liver cirrhosis", *Am-J-Epidemiol*, 1 Dec. 1995, vol. 142 (11), pp. 1136–46, ISSN: 002–9262.

Corrao, G. et al., "Interaction between dietary pattern and alcohol intake on the risk of liver cirrhosis",

Rev-Epidemiol-Santé-Publique 1995, vol. 43(1), pp. 7–17, ISSN: 0398–7620.

D'Amico, G. et al., "Effect of dietary proteins and lipids in patients with membranous nephropathy and nephrotic syndrome", *Clin-Nephrol*, June 1991, vol. 35 (6), pp. 237–42, ISSN: 0301–0430.

Dougall, J. et al., "Rapid reduction of serum cholesterol and blood pressure by a twelve-day, very low fat, strictly vegetarian diet", *J-Am-Coll-Nutr*, Oct. 1995, vol. 14 (5), pp. 491–6, ISSN: 0731–5724.

Eichler, Els., *Wickel und Auflagen (Anleitung für Pflegende)*, 1981, Verein für ein erweitertes Heilwesen e.V., Bad Liebenzell-Unterlengenhardt, 4th expanded edition.

Eppinger, H., "Über Rohkostbehandlung", Vienna, *Klein. Wschr.*, vol. 51, 2nd half year, no. 26, 702–708, 1939.

Eppinger, H., "Einiges über diätetische Therapie", *Ztschr. f. ärztl. Fortbildung*, Verlag Gustav Fischer, Jena, vol. 36, nos. 22 and 23, 673–678, 709–714, 1939.

Everhart. J., "Diet and gallstones in Italy", *Hepatology*, Nov. 1998, vol. 28 (5), pp. 1438–9, ISSN: 0270–9139.

Festi, D. et al., "Gallbladder motility and gallstone formation in obese patients following very low calorie diets. Use it (fat) to loose it (well)", *Int-J-Obes-Relat-Metab-Disord*, June 1998, vol. 22 (6), pp. 592–600, ISSN: 0307–0565.

Friedrich, H. and H. Peters, "Zur Behandlung der Leberzirrhose mit Rohkost", *Münch. Med. Wochenschrift*, vol 86, 1st half year, no. 12, 453–455, 1939.

Gans, R. O. et al., "Fish-oil supplementation in patients with stable claudication", *AM-J-Surg*, Nov. 1990, vol. 160 (5), pp. 490–5, ISSN: 0002–9610.

Gisling, Etzel., *Check up*, No. 6, 1994, p. 4, Infomed-Verlag, Wil.

Gotto, A. M., Jr., "Rationale for treatment", *Am-J-Med*, 31 July 1991, vol. 91 (1B), pp. 315–365, ISSN: 0002–9343 18.

Gupta, R. et al., "Influence of alcohol intake on high density lipoprotein cholesterol levels in middle aged men", *Indian-Heart-J*, May-June 1994, vol. 46 (3), pp. 146–9, ISSN: 0019–4832.

Hahm, J. et al., "Changes in gallbladder motility in gastrectomized patients", *Korean-J-Intern-Med*, Jan. 2000, vol. 15 (1), pp. 19–24, ISSN: 0494–4712.

Harrison, T. R., *Innere Medizin*, German edition from Kurt J. G. Schmailzl, Blackwell Wissenschaftsverlag Berlin, 1995, 13th ed., p. 1762.

Heine, H., "Anatomische Struktur der Akupunkturpunkte", in A. Pischinger, *Das System der Grundregulation. Grundlagen für eine ganzheits-biologische Theorie der Medizin* (1990), 8th ed. Haug-Verlag, Heidelberg.

Heine, H., "Weitreichende Wechselwirkung als Grundlage der Homöostase – funktionelle Aspekte der Neuraltherapie", *Ae-Ztg f. Naturheilverfahren* 28 (1987), p. 915.

Heine, H., "Der Extrazellulärraum – eine vernachlässigte Dimension der Tumorforschung" *Krebsgeschehen* 17, 1985, p. 124.

Heine, H., "Die Grundregulation aus neuer Sicht", *Ae. Ztg. f. Naturheilverfahren* 28, 1987, p. 909.

Heshka, S. et al., "Obesity and risk of gall stone development on a 1200 Kcal/d (5025 Kj/d) regular food diet" (see comments), *Int-J-Obes-Relat-Metab-Disord*, May 1996, vol. 20 (5), pp. 430–4, ISSN: 0307–0565.

Jalovara, P., "Effect of periodic long-term ethanol administration on biliary bile acids and bile secretion in the rat", *Ann-Clin-Res*, 1988, vol. 20 (6), pp. 410–3 ISSN: 0003–4762.

Jung, C. G., "The Concept of the Collective Unconscious" (1936), *Collected Works* vol. 9.I (1959).

Jung, C. G., "Die Beziehungen zwischen dem Ich und dem Unbewussten", Rascher, Zurich, 1933.

Jung, C. G., "Les racines de la conscience", trans. Yves Le Lay et Etienne Perrot, Buchet Chastel, Paris, 1971.

Kaunitz, H., "Transmineralisation und vegetarische Kost", *Ergebn. d. inn. Med. u. Kinderheilk*, Verlag Julius Springer, Berlin, vol. 51, pp. 218–322, 1936.

Keenan, J-M. et al., "Randomised, controlled, crossover trial of oat bran in hyper- cholesterolemic subjects", *J-Fam-Pract*, Dec. 1991, vol. 33 (6), p. 6608, ISSN: 0094–3509.

Kollenbach, D., *Maximilian Oskar Bircher-Benner, Krankheitslehre und Diätetik*, Inaugural Diss., University of Cologne, 21 May 1974, p. 142 .

König, G. and I. Wancura, *Neue chinesische Akupunktur*, Verlag Wilhelm Maudrich, Vienna, Munich, Bern 1989.

Kuhne, Louis., *Die neue Heilwissenschaft*, Verlag der Neuen Heilkunst, Leipzig, 1890.

Kunz, A., "Stoffwechseluntersuchungen bei Bircher-Kost", offprint from *Ergebnisse der physikalisch-diätetischen Therapie*, 315–349, Vol. 3, Arbeitsgemeinschaft med. Verlage, Verlag Theodor Steinkopf, Dresden and Leipzig, 1948.

Laurent, C. et al., "Effect of acetate and propionate on fasting hepatic glucose production in human", *Eur-J-Clin-Nutr*, July 1995, vol. 49 (7), pp. 484–91, ISSN: 0954–3007.

Levin, E. G. et al., "Comparison of psyllium hydrophilic mucilloid and cellulose as adjuncts to prudent diet in the treatment of mild to moderate hypercholesterolemia", *Arch-Int-Med*, Sept. 1990, vol. 150 (9), pp. 1822–7, ISSN: 003–9926.

Li, S. D. et al., "Nutrition support for individuals with liver failure" (clinical conference), 1992, Division of Gastroenterology, Hepatology, and Nutrition, Loyola University Medical Center, Maywood, IL 60183, USA.

Lieber, C. S., "Alcoholic liver disease: new insights in pathogenesis lead to new treatments", *Journal of Hepatology*, 2000, vol. 32 (suppl. 1), pp. 113–28, 189 Refs, ISSN: 0168–8278.

Liechti-v. Brasch, D. and A. Kunz, *Die klinische Bedeutung der Frischkost. Hippokrates, Zeitschrift für praktische Heilung und für die Einheit der Medizin*, Hippokrates-Verlag Stuttgart, 27. ed., Nov. 30, issue 22, pp. 3–11, 1956.

Liechti-v. Brasch, D., "70 Jahre Erfahrungsgut der Bircher-Bennerschen Ordnungstherapie", *Erfahrungsheilkunde*, issue 6, pp. 181–273, 1970.

Liechti-v. Brasch, D., "Rohkostwirkungen", *Diaita* 1979, p. 12.

Melchert, H-U. et al., "Fatty acid pattern in triglycerides, diglycerides, free fatty acids, cholesteryl esters and phosphaticlylcholine in serum from vegetarians and non-vegetarians", *Atherosclerosis*, May 1987, vol. 65 (1–2), pp. 159–66, ISSN: 0021–9150.

Mikhailova, L. P. et al., "Die Uebertragung der Hepatitis B durch Photonen", in Popp, F. A.: *Biologie des Lichtes* (39), Parey-Verlag, Berlin and Heidelberg, 1984.

Mikhailova, L. P. et al., "Ultraschwache Strahlung als interzelluläre Wechselwirkung?" (in Russian), Nauka, Novosibirsk, in Dezowska- Trzebiatowska et al. (eds), *Photon Emission from Biological Systems*, World Scientific, Singapore, New Jersey and Hong Kong, 1986.

Misciagna, G. et al., "Diet, physical activity and gallstones – a population-based, case-control study in Southern Italy", *Am-J-Clin-Nutr*, Jan. 1999, vol. 69 (1), pp. 120–6, ISSN: 0002–9165.

Moerman, C. J. et al., "Consumption of foods and micronutrients and the risk of cancer of the biliary tract", *Prev-Med*, Nov. 1995, vol. 24 (6), pp. 591–602, ISSN: 0091–7435.

Neal, G. W. et al., "Synergetic effects of psyllium in dietary treatment of hyper- cholesterolemia", *South-Med-J*, Oct. 1990, vol. 83 (10), pp. 1131–7, ISSN: 0038–4348.

Nielsen, K. et al., "Long term oral refeeding of patients with cirrhosis of the liver", *B-J-Nutr*, Oct. 1995, vol. 74 (4), pp. 557–67, ISSN: 007–1145.

Noorden, C. von, "Alte und neuzeitliche Ernährungsfragen unter Mitberücksichtigung wirtschaftlicher Gewichts punkte", Julius Springer Verlag, Vienna and Berlin, 1931.

Noorden, C. von, "Ueber Obstkuren und über Rohkost", *Therapie der Gegenwart*, vol. 69, newest series, 30th ed., no. 7, p. 289–298, 1928.

Ornish, D. et al., "Can lifestyle changes reverse coronary heart disease? The Lifestyle Heart Trial" (see comments), *Lancet*, 21 July 1990, vol. 336 (8708), pp. 129–33, ISSN: 0023–7507.

Park, H. S. et al., "Effect of weight control on hepatic abnormalities in obese patients with fatty liver", *J-Korean-Med-S*, Dec. 1995, vol.10 (6), pp. 414–21, ISSN: 1011–8934.

Parker, E. S. et al., "Alcohol and the disruption of cognitive processes", *Arch-Gen-Psychiatry*, Dec. 1974, vol. 31 (6), pp. 824–8, ISSN: 0003–990X.

Pischinger, A. et al., *Das System der Grundregulation. Grundlagen für eine ganzheits-biologische Theorie der Medizin*, (1990), 8th ed., Haug-Verlag, Heidelberg.

Portincasa, P. et al., "Gallbladder motility and cholesterol crysiallisation in bile from patients with pigment and cholesterol gallstones", *Eur-J-Clin-Invest*, April 2000, vol. 30 (4), pp. 317–24, ISSN: 0014–2972.

Rich, H. G., "Resolution of focal fatty in-filtration of the liver", *South-Med-J*, Oct. 1996, vol. 89 (10), pp. 1024–7 Refs, ISSN: 0038–4348.

Ritter, M. M. et al., "Effects of vegetarian lifestyle on health", *Fortschritt-Med*, 10 June 1995, vol. 113 (16), pp. 239–42, ISSN: 0015–8178.

Rottka, H., "Health and vegetarian lifestyle", *Bibl.-Nutr-Pieta*, 1990 (45), pp. 176–194, ISSN: 0067–8198, 66 Refs.

Ruhl, C. E. and J. E. Everhart, "Association of diabetes, serum insulin, and C-peptide with gallbladder disease" (see comments), Hepatology, Feb. 2000, vol. 31 (2), pp. 299–303, ISSN: 0276–9139.

Sciarrone, S. E. et al., "A factorial study of salt restriction and a low-fat/high-fibre diet in hypertensive subjects", *J-Hypertens*, Mar. 1992, vol. 10 (3), pp. 287–98, ISSN: 0263–6352.

Shepard, R. W., "Pre- and postoperative nutritional care in liver transplantation in children", *J-Gastroenterol-Hepatol*, May 1996, vol. 11 (5), R: 57–10, ISSN: 0815–9319.

Sherman, D. I. et al., "Safe drinking limits?" (letter), *Addiction*, Feb. 1994, vol. 89 (2), pp. 235, ISSN: 0965–2140.

Simsek, H. et al., "Effect of prolonged ethanol intake on pancreatic lipids in the rat pancreas", *Pancreas*, July 1990, vol. 5 (4), pp. 401–7, ISSN: 0885–3177.

Singh, R-B. et al., "Randomised controlled trial of cardioprotective diet in patients with recent acute myocardial infarction: results of one year follow up", *BMJ*, 18 Apr. 1992, vol. 304 (6833), pp. 1015–9, ISSN 0959–8138.

Skuladottir, G. V. et al., "Influence of dietary cod liver oil on fatty acid composition of plasma lipids in human male subjects after myocardial infarction", *J-Intern-Med*, Dec. 1990, vol. 228 (6), pp. 563–8, ISSN: 0954–6820.

Socha, P. et al., "Essential fatty add metabolism in infants with cholelithiasis", *Acta-Pediatr*, Mar. 1998, vol. 87 (3), pp. 278–83, ISSN: 0803–5253.

Spengler, Wilhelm, *Kneipplehre und Naturheilung*, Turm-Verlag, Bietigheim/Württ., 1969, p. 712.

Stehelin, H. B., "Critical rappraisal of vitamins and trace minerals in nutritional support for cancer patients", *Support-Care-Cancer*, Nov. 1993, vol. 1 (6), pp. 295–97, ISSN: 0941–4355.

Tandon, R. K. et al., "Dietary habits of gall- stone patients in Northern India", *J-Clin-Gastroenterology*, Jan. 1996, vol. 22 (1), pp. 23–7, ISSN: 0192–0790.

Thomas, L. A. et al., "Mechanism for the transit-induced increase in colonic deoxycholic acid formation in cholesterol cholelithiasis", *Gastroenterology*, Sept. 2000, vol. 119 (3), pp. 806–15, ISSN: 0016–5085.

Thüler, Maya., *Wohltuende Wickel*, 5th ed. January 1993, copyright 1986, 1993 by Maya Thüler Verlag, Schmitteplatz 18, CH-3076 Worb, ISBN: 3–908539-01-3.

Tseng, M. et al., "Food intake patterns and gallbladder disease in Mexican Americans", *Public-Health-Nutr*, June 2000, vol. 3 (2) pp. 233–43, ISSN: 1368–9800.

Tsugare, S. et al., "Alcohol consumption and all-cause and cancer mortality among middle-aged Japanese men: seven-year follow-up of the JPIIC study, Cohort I, Japan Public Health Center", *American Journal of Epidemiology*, Dec. 1, 1999, Vol 150 (11), pp. 1201–07, ISSN: 0002–9262.

Ueno, T. et al., "Therapeutic effects of restricted diet and exercise in obese patients with fatty liver", *J-Hepatol*, July 1997, vol. 27 (1), pp. 103–7, ISSN: 0168–8278.

Vezina, W. C., "Similarity in gallstone for- mation from 900 Kcal/day diets containing main culprit of cholelithiasis during rapid weight reduction," *Dig-Dis-Sci*, Mar. 1998, vol. 43 (3), pp. 554–61, ISSN: 0163–2116.

Voytechovsky, M. et al., "The influence of alcohol on memory functions in healthy volunteers", *Act-Nerv-Saper* (Prague), 1970, vol. 12 (3), pp. 255–6.

Waagh, M. et al., "Effect of social drinking on neuropsychological performance", *Br-J-Addict*, June 1989, vol. 84 (6), pp. 659–67, ISSN: 0952–0481.

Wannametzee, G. et al., "Alcohol and sudden cardiac death", 1992, a paper of the Department of Public Health and Primary Care, Royal Free Hospital School of Medicine, London NW32 PF.

Watanabe, A. et al., "Nutrient induced thermogenesis and protein sparing effect by rapid infusion of a branched chain enriched amino acid solution to cirrhotic patients", *J-Med*, 1996, vol. 27 (3–4), pp. 176–82, ISSN: 0025–7850.

Watts, G. F. et al., "Effects on coronary artery disease of lipid-lowering diet, or diet plus cholestyramine, in the St Thomas' Atherosclerosis Regression Study (STARS)", *Lancet*, 7 Mar 1992, vol. 339 (8793) pp. 563–9, ISSN: 0023–7507.

Webster, P. D. et al., "Secretory and metabolic effects of alcohol on the pancreas", *Ann-N-Y-Acad-Sci*, 25 Apr. 1975, vol. 252, pp. 183–6, ISSN: 0077–8923 9.

Whitby, K. E. et al., "Developmental effects of combined exposure to ethanol and vitamin A",

Food-Chem-Toxicol, Apr. 1994, vol. 32 (4), pp. 305–20, ISSN: 0278–6915.

White, J-L. et al., "Oat bran lowers plasma cholesterol levels in mildly hypercholesterolemic men", *J-Am-Diet-Assoc*, Apr. 1992, vol. 92 (4), pp. 446–9, ISSN: 0002–8223.

Winternitz, Wilhelm, *Die Hydrotherapie auf physiologischer und klinischer Grundlage*, Urban & Schwarzenberg, Vienna, 1877.

Wood, P. D., "The effects an plasma kipo- proteins of a prudent weight-reducing diet, with or without exercise in overweight men and women", *N-Engl-J-Med*, 15 Aug. 1991, vol. 325 (7), pp. 461–6, ISSN: 0028–4793.

Yinnon, A. M. et al., "A Practical Intervention Programme Aimed at Decreasing High Serum Cholesterol Levels in Primary Care", *Fam-Pract*, Jan. 1992, vol. 9 (2), pp. 167–70, ISSN: 0263–2136.

Zapata, R. et al., "Gallbladder motility and lithogenesis in obese patients during diet-induced weight loss", *Dig-Dis-Sci*, Feb. 2000, vol. 45 (2), pp. 421–8, ISSN: 0163–2116.

Zippelius, 1999 (page 20)

Index

Adiposity	12, 18, 19		Fatty acid profile	19
Alcohol	21, 22, 28		Fatty liver	20, 28
Amanita poisoning	28			
Ascites	18, 28		Gallbladder carcinoma	32
Australia-Antigen	26		Gallbladder colic	30
			Gallbladder inflammation	30
Basic substance of			Gallbladder inflammation,	
the soft connective tissue	10		chronic	31
Bile-duct stones	32		Gallstones	30
Bleeding tendency	28			
Breathing, conscious	54		Haemorrhoids	12, 13, 28
Brucella	27		Healing crisis	56, 57
Butter, plant and			Healing regime	50
vegetable fats and oils	72		Heart-attack risk	12, 19
			Hepatitis	25
Casein protein	16		Hepatitis A	26
Cholangitis	32		Hepatitis B	26
Cholecystectomy	49		Hepatitis C	27
Cholecystitis-treatment	53		Hepatitis D	27
Choledocholithiasis	32		Hepatitis E	27
Cholesterol	12		Hepatitis, infectious	26
Circadian rhythm	24, 53		Hepatitis, toxic and	
Cirrhotic liver (liver cirrhosis)	28		medication	27
Colitis (inflammation of the			Hepatitis-treatment	27
large intestine)	25		Homeopathy	44
Coronary sclerosis	12, 20, 23		Hyperplasia, focal nodular	29
Cravings, paradoxical	25			
Cycle, enterohepatic	12		Inflammation of the	
			large intestine (Colitis)	25
Depression	26, 47, 57		Interference field	47
Diet Stage I	56		Interferon a	27
Diet Stage II	58		Intestinal regulation	25, 52
Diet stage III	59		Intestinal symbiosis	18
Diet stage IV	62			
			Jaundice	25, 26, 32
Echinococcus (tapeworms)	27			
Encephalopathy, hepatic	29		Liver adenoma	29
Enterohepatic cycle	12		Liver carcinoma	29
Epstein-Barr virus	27		Liver cirrhosis	28
			Liver cirrhosis treatment	52
			Liver failure	25, 29

Liver metastases	30	Regulation block	48
Liver transplant	49		
		Secondary phenomenon	48
Membrane potential	47, 50	Spagyrics	34
Mononucleosis	27	Stress, miasmatic	45
		Substitution table for animal products	63
Neural therapy	47, 48		
Occlusion icterus	32	Toxoplasmosis	27
Oesophageal varices	28	Treatment of infections	35
Oils, butter and vegetable fats	72	Triglycerides	19
Omega-3-fatty acids	19		
		Uric-acid level of the blood	12
Postcholecystectomy syndrome	32, 48, 49	Vegetable fats, Butter and oils	72

CENTRE FOR SCIENTIFIC NATURAL MEDICINE

People come to the Bircher-Benner Medical Centre from a large number of countries in search of healing.

Here, you will be valued as a unique person, listened to and understood. Here, humanity and dignity are important and the medicine is a noble undertaking.

Centre for scientific natural medicine

Our fresh-vegetable diet will bring about a rapid change in your metabolism; natural regulative therapies take precedence where possible.

The atmosphere and the living tradition of the Bircher-Benner Centre, where novelty and modernity are combined with decades of experience, contribute to your healing.

The doctors and therapists will treat you personally and have all the facilities of a modern clinic at hand when needed.

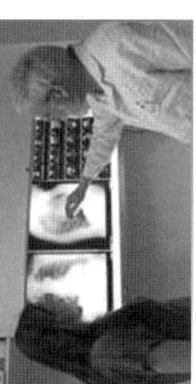

The search for the true causes of diseases is central to our work, as is the inclusion of your self-curative powers in the process of healing.

The supplementation of traditional medicine by the regulative diagnosis and therapy of natural healing often permits a cure where the usual therapies have failed.

In the Medical Centre, you can relax and recover, and will experience the deep regeneration of your healing powers.

CENTRE BIRCHER-BENNER
CH-8784 Braunwald

Phone: +41 (0)21 801 60 04
Fax: +41 (0)55 643 16 93
info@bircher-benner.com
www.bircher-benner.com

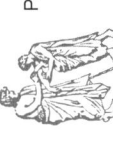

Indications: any internal diseases, migraine, tinnitus, neuralgia and other pain conditions, fibromyalgia, arthritis and arthrosis, collagenoses, liver, gallbladder and gastrointestinal diseases, metabolic diseases and diabetes, cardiovascular diseases, kidney and prostate diseases, women's diseases, allergies, skin diseases, convalescence, fatigue, depression and anxiety, menopausal, hormonal and weight problems.